# the GI counter

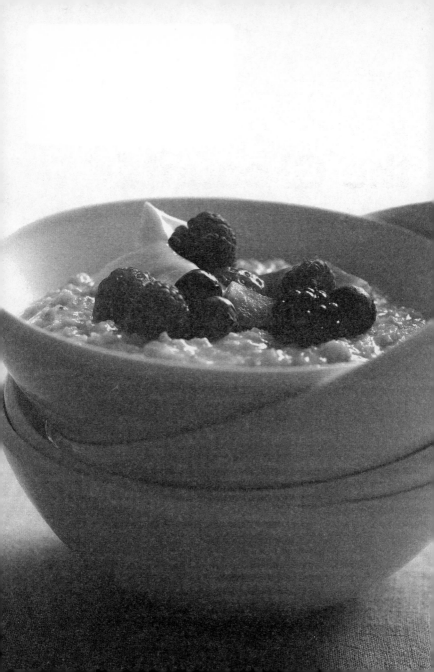

Dr Mabel Blades

# the **GI** counter

GI values for almost 1000 foods at a glance

with a foreword by **Anthony Worrall Thompson**

Kyle Cathie Ltd

# acknowledgements

Many thanks to all the food producers and nutritionists who
provided information for this book, to my editor Caroline Taggart,
to Antony Worrall Thompson for his foreword and to my husband
Peter for all his help and support.

First published in Great Britain in 2007 by
Kyle Cathie Limited
122 Arlington Road
London NW1 7HP
general.enquiries@kyle-cathie.com
www.kylecathie.com

10 9 8 7 6 5 4 3 2

ISBN 978 1 85626 719 9

Edited by Caroline Taggart
Design by Geoff Hayes

A Cataloguing in Publication record for this title is available from the
British Library

Printed and bound in Great Britain by Cox and Wyman

# contents

# foreword by
# Antony Worrall Thompson

I am a great believer in GI. I first found out about it a few years ago when I was diagnosed with Syndrome X, a pre-diabetic condition that meant it was suddenly vital that I lose weight, keep an eye on my blood sugar and take a lot more care about my diet. For ever. I love good food and the prospect of having to eat less and feel perpetually hungry filled me with gloom. On top of that, I knew from many years of being overweight that most diets are so boring that only a saint can stick to them for any length of time.

I needn't have worried. The beauty of the GI diet is that, although you do have to cut down on a few indulgences, everything you eat is immensely satisfying. You don't crave a bar of chocolate in the middle of the morning, because your breakfast is still keeping you going. And you don't have those rushes of blood to the head that make you feel high after lunch, then miserable and sluggish around four o'clock. Once I discovered this, I developed my own low-GI diet – and wrote a book about it – to help other people change their habits for life.

I am also a great believer in Dr Mabel Blades. As a highly qualified and experienced dietitian and nutritionist, she helped me enormously with *Antony Worrall Thompson's GI Diet*. But that is largely a recipe book, and nobody can try new recipes all the time. We need to know more about the GI values of the foods we see every day on our supermarket shelves, and that is what Mabel's GI Counter provides. Research into GI values is in its infancy, and it is an extraordinary achievement on Mabel's part to have produced the detailed figures in this book. It is a huge step forward in enabling all of us to make informed decisions about the food we buy.

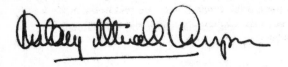

# introduction

The Glycaemic Index or GI is the value given to different 'carbohydrate foods' based on the impact that each food has on blood-sugar levels.

There are many reasons why you might want to keep an eye on your GI intake, and this counter has been developed to help you choose food wisely rather than having to look at lots of other lists, websites and packs. And, because carbohydrate content or GI should not be considered in isolation, I have also provided information on calorie content, fat and sodium levels.

### WHAT ARE CARBOHYDRATE FOODS?

**Carbohydrate is the term used for those foods, which contain a large proportion of carbohydrate. There are two main types of carbohydrate – the sugars and the starches.**

**The sugary carbohydrates are (obviously) those foods which contain a lot of sugar, such as jam, cakes, sweet biscuits, sweets, chocolate and many soft drinks. Starchy foods contain a large proportion of starch and include bread, pasta, rice, potatoes, breakfast cereals and noodles.**

**However, carbohydrate foods are not made up exclusively of carbohydrate – they may well contain other nutrients such as protein, fibre, vitamins, minerals and fat, as well as water. For example white bread – classified as a 'carbohydrate food' – consists of approximately 46% carbohydrate, 8% protein, 2% fibre, 2% fat and 39% water, with the rest being made up of minerals such as calcium, iron, zinc and sodium and the B vitamin group.**

### So what exactly is GI?

The Glycaemic Index measures the way in which we break down carbohydrate foods into the simple sugar glucose, which is then absorbed and used in our bodies for energy. Foods with a low GI sustain our blood sugar levels, or rather blood glucose levels, for longer than those with a high GI, which cause a peak in blood sugar levels followed by a slump. When our blood sugars are maintained at a moderate level we tend not to feel hungry. When the level zooms up after eating a high GI food, the dramatic dip that follows takes blood sugars down to a level at which we can feel really hungry.

It must be emphasised that the GI is concerned solely with carbohydrates, so protein foods and fats all have 0 GI, because they are not made up of glucose units. This fact has led to some controversy about the value of a low GI diet, but in my experience most people who are trying to lose weight, or are keeping an eye on their diet for specific health reasons, are sensible enough to know that fats are high in calories and that too many lead to weight gain!

## CALORIES FROM NUTRIENTS

**All foods and beverages (with the exception of water) provide energy – calories (normally measured as kilocalories, which means thousands of calories, hence the abbreviation kcal).**

**Carbohydrate provides 3.75kcal per gram**
**Protein provides 4kcal per gram**
**Fat provides 9kcal per gram**
**Alcohol provides 7kcal per gram**

**To lose weight we need to consume more calories than we take in, which means reducing the overall calorie content of the food we eat and increasing activity so that the body uses up the stores of fat.**

**An average woman requires 2000kcal per day and a man 2500. To lose weight we need to reduce our daily calorie intake by about 500kcal to 1500kcal for a woman and 2000kcal for a man. This will give a slow but steady weight loss of about 0.5-1kg per week.**

**But although many people are obsessed with their weight and trying to lose it, they really should be trying to lose body fat while preserving muscle tissue by including exercise in their daily pattern.**

Research on the GI values of foods began in the 1970s and was further developed in the 1980s as a way of helping those with diabetes to control their condition. GI has since moved to the forefront of nutritional research, especially in Australia, where it has become an increasingly popular method of weight control.

Most of the research is based on giving volunteers the amount of a food that contains 50g of carbohydrate and, by taking blood sugar samples, comparing their blood sugar response to what happens when they take 50g of pure glucose. As human responses vary from individual to individual, there may be some small variation in results – but, like everything else in nutrition, this is not an exact science and a GI point either way will not make much difference to a diet.

Because the carbohydrate contents of foods vary, the volunteers have to eat different quantities of each food. For example, while a large baguette weighing approximately 100g would provide 50g of carbohydrate, you would have to munch your way through 4 apples (approximately 400g) to get the same amount of carbohydrate.

Also, with some foods you would have to eat or drink vast quantities in order to get the 50g of carbohydrate required for testing, so these items have not been tested and are often assigned a very low GI. A good example of this is various alcoholic drinks: it is realistic to test beers, as they contain around 2g carbohydrate per 100ml, which equates to about 10g carbohydrate in half a pint of beer. This means that volunteers would have to drink 2-3 pints in order to take in the required 50g of carbohydrate. Wine, however, contains less than 0.5g carbohydrate per 100ml, so they would have to drink over 10 litres in order to comply with the requirements of the test. You would end up with some extremely tipsy and probably very ill volunteers – which is hardly in line with the ethics of nutritional science.

Many herbs and green vegetables also contain very small amounts of carbohydrate, which makes testing difficult, so again they are considered to have a negligible GI.

Another variation is that some researchers have used white bread rather than glucose as the standard against which to make comparisons, which may be the reason for GI values over 100.

## A WORD OF WARNING

**Do be sure to view GI figures with a little caution, as they differ from variety to variety of, for example, rice, fruit or vegetables and from recipe to recipe with different brands of made-up products such as jams or breakfast cereals.**

**Wherever possible, I have tried to find the precise GI values for foods. A number of other writers have allocated only a low, medium or high GI – although this is helpful, I feel that more accurate information helps you to make more informed choices. For example, as noted below, 'low GI' can be anything up to 55, so there is a big difference between a food that has a GI of 5 and one with a GI of 50.**

### Conditions helped by a low GI diet

A diet with a low GI is considered to be helpful in a number of conditions, including:

● *Managing weight loss and preventing weight gain* by promoting a feeling of fullness and avoiding the very low blood sugar levels which send you running for a snack.

● *Diabetes*, because it helps stabilise blood sugar levels.

● *Raised cholesterol levels*, as the soluble fibres found in such low GI foods as oats and fruit and vegetables reduce the absorption of saturated fat and cholesterol – see the box opposite for more about the different types of fibre.

● *Polycystic ovary syndrome (PCOS)*, from which increasing numbers of women (some say as many as 10-15%) are found to suffer and in which a maintenance of the blood sugar is important. Symptoms of PCOS include irregular or absent periods, very greasy skin, facial hair growth, hair loss, mood swings and difficulties with excessive weight gain.

● *Metabolic syndrome* (sometimes referred to as syndrome X), which is the pre-condition for Type 2 diabetes and coronary heart disease. It is characterised by weight gain (especially around the middle area, giving the so-called 'apple shape'), raised blood pressure, high blood sugar and high cholesterol levels, as well as raised triglyceride levels (see next entry).

● *Raised triglyceride levels*, which can contribute to coronary heart disease in a similar way to raised cholesterol levels.

● *Improving behaviour in young people*, due to the sustained energy levels which help concentration and good behaviour.

● *Digestive problems such as irritable bowel syndrome*, because the diet includes more fibre and promotes a healthy bacterial population in the digestive tract.

● *Constipation*, which is often due to too little fibre and fluid in the diet. Although people don't tend to talk about this, it is both common and unpleasant. A low GI diet with its generous amounts of vegetables and fruit (and hence fibre), as well as plenty of fluid, can be of great assistance in relieving the problem.

● *Low blood sugar levels (hypoglycaemia)* can be helped by the sustained blood sugar levels that frequent snacks of low GI foods bring.

### A NOTE ABOUT FIBRE

**Dietary fibre used to be known as roughage and is scientifically known as non-starch polysaccharide (NSP). It is found only in plant foods such as cereals, fruit and vegetables. The body cannot use it for energy, so in humans its purpose is to add bulk to the diet. It is, however, the main source of energy for ruminant animals like sheep and cows.**

*There are two types of fibre:*
**Soluble fibre is found mainly in oats, barley, fruit and vegetables, especially dried vegetables such as lentils, split peas and beans.**

**Insoluble fibre is found mainly in wheat products such as bread, pasta and breakfast cereals.**

**Soluble fibre is important in moderating blood cholesterol and blood sugar levels, while insoluble fibre is particularly beneficial for bowel health.**

**Both types are filling, so eating plenty of foods containing fibre, especially fruit and vegetables, really helps to fill you up.**

### Low, medium and high GI foods

Carbohydrate foods are the source of energy that all cells of our body can easily use. They are also the only source of energy for our brains. As already seen, they are a less concentrated source of energy than fats, alcohol or protein. This means that we can eat more of them to get the same amount of calories, which is good news for those with big appetites.

Carbohydrates are divided into two main groups, sugars and starches, but during the process of digestion and absorption both are broken down into the tiny molecules of sugars of which they are composed. It is this sugar that is absorbed into the bloodstream.

The predominant sugar which circulates in our blood is the simple sugar glucose and this is derived mainly from starchy carbohydrates such as bread, pasta, breakfast cereals, rice, potatoes, cous cous, biscuits and crackers. 'Complex' sugars such as table sugar (properly known as sucrose) also have a component of glucose, as does the sugar in milk (lactose) and malt, which is used in flavourings for such foods as breakfast cereals.

Various factors affect the GI of a carbohydrate food. These include:

● The way the food is prepared e.g. fruit juice has a higher GI than whole fruit, as in making it you lose the fibres which slow down the absorption of glucose. Another good reason for eating plenty of fresh fruit.

● The structure of the starch and sugars – different varieties of the same food may contain different types of starch, so may have a different GI. Plain boiled potatoes of the variety Desiree, for example, have a higher GI than many other potatoes cooked in the same way. Indeed plant breeders are working on food crops such as potatoes and rice to produce varieties with a lower GI.

● Tough fibrous coatings such as are found in seeds. These have to be broken down during digestion, which means they take more time to be attacked in the digestive process and thus they have a low GI.

● Soluble fibres such as are found in oats, lentils and barley. These slow down the digestion, giving these foods a low GI.

● Reheating. With some carbohydrate foods this can change the structure of the starch, which is why tinned potatoes, bought ready cooked and then reheated, have a lower GI than ordinary boiled ones. However, freshly cooked foods retain more of the vitamins.

● Mixing low GI carbohydrate foods with those with a higher GI in a meal or snack lowers the overall GI of the mixture.

● Adding foods which contain zero GI such as fat or protein to a meal will reduce the GI (but note the warning above about eating too much fat).

### SO WHAT IS 'LOW GI'?

**A 'low GI' is classified as 55 or below. Low GI foods include oats, apples, leafy vegetables and lentils.**

**A 'medium GI' is 56-69. Medium GI foods include carrots, melon, crumpets and pitta bread.**

**A 'high GI' is 70 or above. High GI foods include bagels, white rice, dates and jacket potatoes.**

### Fats
These have a GI of 0, as they contain no carbohydrate. But they are all high in calories, with 9kcal per gram. So fat intake needs to be limited in a healthy diet.

**Mono-unsaturates** such as olive oil and rapeseed oil are the fats suggested for health.

**Polyunsaturates**, found in soya and corn oil, are also considered to be beneficial.

**Omega-3 fatty acids** are essential for brain development and function as well as general health, as they are associated with lower levels of coronary heart disease. They are found mainly in oily fish (see page 20).

**Saturated fats**, found in dairy products such as butter, hard margarine, lard and cream, are considered to be more harmful to health, so use these sparingly.

### Fruit and vegetables

We should eat at least five portions of fruit and vegetables each day. This is about 400g in total. (Remember that potatoes are classed as a starchy food and do not count towards the five portions). Not only are fruit and vegetables generally low in calories but they also contain those all-important protective substances of antioxidants and fibre.

#### WHAT IS 'A PORTION'?

**As a rough guide (remember this is not an exact science!), a portion is:**

- **a medium-sized apple, peach, banana or pear**
- **half a large fruit such as a grapefruit**
- **2 plums**
- **a slice of melon, mango, or pineapple**
- **a teacup or handful of berries or grapes**
- **3 tablespoons of tinned or stewed fruit**
- **dried fruit also counts and a portion is about the same amount as if the fruit were fresh e.g. 3 dried apricots, 2 dried figs or a handful of raisins or sultanas**
- **a small glass or carton of fruit juice – this only counts as one portion per day no matter how much is taken, as the fibre is removed in the process of making juice**
- **a cereal-bowlful of salad**
- **3 tablespoons of cooked vegetable**
- **a handful of raw vegetable sticks**

### Using this counter

Obtaining information on the GI of foods is not easy, as I have found in compiling this book! I have spent many a frustrating hour looking at information from various research establishments from around the world and then scouring supermarkets and shops as I tried to link these up with foods available in the UK. I contacted a number of dietetic colleagues, researchers from major supermarkets, food producers and organisations that produced special products such as those aimed at slimmers. Unfortunately most were unable to help as their organisation did not (yet) undertake the analysis for GI.

For those manufacturers that do provide information on the GI of their products – such as the Alpro dairy-free range, Fuisana, who produce sugars, and Mountain Breads (produced by an Australian company) – I have given specifics, but they are few and far between.

Where information is available, values for the same food may vary from one list to another because the research has been done on different varieties of fruit or vegetables, or in different countries, where even what we know as staple foods may have different compositions and recipes. For the purposes of this book, common values have been taken and some estimates made based on averages.

Sometimes packs provide information on the Glycaemic Load (GL, see below) rather than the GI (as with the Nairn oat cakes), so in these instances I have done the calculations required to convert the figures to GI values.

### GLYCAEMIC LOAD (GL)

**The Glycaemic Load is a development of the Glycaemic Index that takes into account the amount of carbohydrate in a food and the body's response to it as well as its GI.**

**The GL is calculated by multiplying the amount of carbohydrate in a normal-sized portion of the food by the GI of the food and then dividing by 100.**

**So, for example, baked beans in tomato sauce have an average GI of 48, which counts as low. An average 100g portion contains 15g of carbohydrate, so the GL is 48 x 15 = 720, divided by 100, thus the GL is 7, which is also low.**

**However, this means doing a fairly complicated calculation for each food, whereas the GI exists as an established measure. Where the GL comes into its own is with a food such as watermelon, of which you would have to eat a vast amount in order to take in 50g of carbohydrate. It has a GI rating of 72 (high), but if you take an average portion size of 150g, you get a**

**GL of only 8. It's one of those areas where using your common sense and taking calorie count and portion size into account will take you a long way.**

**But as a guide for those who want to know more about GL levels:**

**Low 0–10**
**Medium 11–19**
**High 20+**

In general a woman wanting to lose weight on 1500kcal per day should eat about 200g of carbohydrate, and a man trying to lose weight on 2000kcal per day about 260g. At least half of this should have a low GI i.e. below 55.
The main point is to try to keep mostly to low GI carbohydrate foods. That means lots of fresh foods like fruit and vegetables – which we all know are the basis of a healthy diet. It is also sensible to combine carbohydrate foods with a protein food such as meat, fish, eggs or cheese or vegetable sources of proteins such as pulses or nuts. For flavour and ease in cooking perhaps add a little healthy fat like olive oil or rapeseed oil.

Obviously you need to be sensible as to portion sizes, as massive meals will not help anyone to lose weight!

This type of low GI diet makes a sensible, balanced eating programme which will keep you feeling full and energetic, as well as providing all the nutrients needed for health.

**Other Nutritional Information**
To help you make choices on how to fit 'low GI' into other aspects of a healthy diet, I have given calorie counts and also information on the fat, carbohydrate and sodium content of foods. These nutrients are all detailed in amounts per 100g, so they tie in with the information provided on food pack labels.

Again remember that the values of these nutrients can vary with different brands from different manufacturers, so if you are comparing pack information you may see some slight discrepancies.

*Calories*
Knowing the calorie count of a food enables you to choose between different protein foods, which all have a GI of 0, and is obviously useful for anyone who is trying to avoid gaining weight, to lose weight or to maintain a new lower weight and lower body fat percentage.

Controlling portion sizes is another sensible way to avoid taking in excessive calories and fat (see below).

Remember that losing weight should always be done slowly, no more than 0.5–1kg a week if you expect to keep the weight off. Indeed what you really should be trying to do is lose body fat and acquire more lean body mass as you get fitter and develop more muscles. If you are severely overweight and your weight is soaring, it may be worth trying to maintain it for a week by eating sensibly, choosing plenty of low GI carbohydrates as well as doing more exercise such as walking. If you do not manage to control your eating habits and stop gaining weight, it is unlikely that you will be able to stick to a weight-loss eating pattern and maintain a new lower weight; in this case you may be well advised to consult your doctor for further assistance and perhaps a referral to a registered dietitian.

### SUGGESTED PORTION SIZES FOR PROTEIN FOODS

**100–150g raw weight of meat, poultry or fish – this means a piece about the size of a pack of cards**
**25–30g cheese – around the size of a matchbox, which looks a lot more and goes further if it is grated**
**2 medium eggs**

**As nuts, seeds, and pulses have some carbohydrate in them they have a GI figure which is seen in the list. Nuts and seeds also contain fat and are therefore relatively high in calories. So they need to be limited to portions of around 25g rather than nibbled by the handful if you are trying to lose weight.**

**Pulses have a low GI and also are relatively low in calories, so have portion sizes of about 100–200g. These foods are brilliant in dishes such as casseroles and curries to give added bulk as well as extra flavour.**

*Carbohydrate*
Watching carbohydrate intake is particularly important for those with diabetes, but may also be sensible for some women with polycystic ovary syndrome (PCOS). People of either sex who have raised triglycerides (a sticky substance which can be found in the blood and which can clog up the arteries in a way similar to the harmful type of cholesterol) may also be advised to limit the amount of sugary carbohydrates that they eat.

*Fat*

Fat is higher in calories than carbohydrates, protein and even alcohol (see box on page 22). For many people, reducing the amount of fat in the diet reduces overall calorie intake and hence helps with weight loss. Excess fat – particularly of the saturated type found in animal products such as lard, full-cream milk and cheese, butter and the fat on meat – is also linked with coronary heart disease, so a knowledge of the fat content of foods can assist those with this problem as well as those who are watching their fat intake for other reasons.

Saturated fat is also found in foods such as pastry, cakes, creamy sauces, hard margarine and coconut cream and oil. (Beware of these last two – many people are amazed to see how much saturated fat there is in dishes such as Thai-style curries using these ingredients.)

We all need some fat in our diet for maintenance of the brain and nervous tissues, and as a base for making some hormones and vitamin D. This book allows you to choose fats like those from oils and oily fish to provide these (see page 20 for a list of 'oily fish').

*Sodium*

The chemical name for salt is sodium chloride, and sodium is the damaging component found in it. Anyone with high blood pressure or heart problems is likely to be advised by their doctor to limit their sodium levels, but today we are all encouraged to reduce the amount of salt we eat.

To work out the amount of salt in a food from the sodium figures given in this book, multiply by 2.5. i.e. 1g of sodium is present in 2.5g of salt. Adults are recommended to have no more than 6g of salt (2.4g of sodium) per day.

The Food Standards Agency has been working hard to inform the public about salt in food and to encourage them to cut it down. They have also been encouraging food manufacturers to reduce the salt content in their products. This is probably one of the reasons why so few manufacturers have yet turned their attention to research into GI.

**How foods are listed**

Foods included in this book are divided into categories such as fruit, vegetables and dairy products, and arranged in an order that roughly imitates your progress through the supermarket. But as some foods are thought of by different people in different groupings, a few have been listed twice. For example, in the 'Balance of Good Health', which is the illustration of a healthy balanced diet advocated by the Food Standards Agency, potatoes are grouped with starchy carbohydrate foods like bread, pasta and rice. However, many people think of them as vegetables and this is where they are found in the supermarket. So for 'correctness' and ease of use, potatoes are listed on their own. Similarly, in the 'Balance of Good Health', butter is considered a fat, but many people consider it a dairy food, so it is listed in both sections.

We have tried hard to make the print easy to read, and the vibrant pink cover has been chosen to help you find the book at the bottom of your handbag!

### Fitting 'low GI' into a healthy eating plan
The following are the Food Standards Agency's eight tips for making healthier choices:

1 Base your meals on starchy foods
2 Eat lots of fruit and vegetables
3 Eat more fish – including a portion of oily fish each week
4 Cut down on saturated fat and sugar
5 Try to eat less salt – no more than 6g a day for adults
6 Get active and try to be a healthy weight
7 Drink plenty of water
8 Don't skip breakfast

*Base your meals on starchy foods*
These foods should make up about a third of your daily intake. Starchy foods are major sources of energy, B vitamins and dietary fibre.

This is easy to achieve on a low GI diet – it just means a few substitutions. For example, use thick slices of wholegrain seeded bread or grain breads instead of white, brown or wholemeal in your sandwiches. These breads also make delicious toast, as well as being satisfying in bread puddings.

Use more small potatoes boiled in their skins instead of mashed or jacket potatoes, or serve jacket potatoes with a low GI food such as baked beans, to reduce the overall GI level.

Swap white rice for brown basmati, which has the lowest GI of any rice, and include more pasta dishes on your menu.

Try adding low GI items like barley to your soup or experiment with bulgar wheat in casseroles or as an alternative to rice or potatoes.

*Eat lots of fruit and vegetables*
As a nation we are still not eating those all-important five portions of fruit and vegetables each day.

A low GI diet really encourages the inclusion of more vegetables, as most have a low GI, so they reduce the overall GI of a meal. Vegetables are also low in fat, low in salt and low in calories – lots of good reasons for eating plenty of them!

Fresh vegetables obviously have more flavour – especially if newly harvested from the garden. But these days a range of frozen, tinned and 'ready to steam' vegetables is available too, so there is no excuse for not including more vegetables on the grounds that you haven't got time to prepare them. While tinned and dried vegetables will have lost vitamins during their processing, frozen ones have the vitamins safely locked in so are probably the best alternative to fresh. If you choose tinned vegetables, look at the sodium content and go for those without added salt.

Using a steamer or microwave in which vegetables can be cooked in minutes is the best way to preserve flavour and colour. Also vegetables and pulses can be added to a casserole in a slow cooker which brings out the full flavour.

Many fruits, especially apples, bananas, cherries, plums and berries, also have a low GI. They make excellent snacks and additions to cereals, and bananas are great in sandwiches. Fruit is also the perfect accompaniment to ice creams and yoghurts. And, like vegetables, it is generally low in calories, fat and sodium.

Having been deeply immersed in looking at information on nutrition and GI in the course of preparing this book, if there is one thing I want to emphasise it is eat more vegetables. They contain many protective nutrients, they are low in calories and fat, wonderful for flavour and generally inexpensive.

*Eat more fish – including a portion of oily fish each week*
Fish, like all protein food, has a GI of 0, so it makes a good combination with high-GI foods. Avoid frying it, especially in batter or breadcrumbs, to keep the fat content down.

Salmon, mackerel, trout, herrings, fresh tuna, sardines, pilchards and eel are all classed as oily fish, and therefore good sources of Omega-3 fatty acids (see above). They can be combined with potatoes or pasta and vegetables in various hot dishes, or eaten hot or cold with salad.

*Cut down on saturated fat and sugar*
Cutting down on saturated fat is associated with promoting heart health. When looking at the fat content figures given in this book, bear in mind that 20g or more of fat per 100g in a food is generally considered 'a lot' and 3g or less is 'a little'. A lot of saturated fat is 5g per 100g of food and a little is 1g per 100g. Sugar is associated with dental decay when eaten too frequently. 10g of sugar per 100g of food represents high sugar content, and 2g per 100g is low.

*Try to eat less salt — no more than 6g a day for adults*
Most of our salt intake comes from manufactured foods and as a low GI diet is based on lots of fresh foods like vegetables and fruit it should be relatively easy to keep below the 6g guideline.

When it comes to salt, 1.25g of salt or 0.5g of sodium per 100g of food is regarded as a lot. A low level of salt is 0.25g of salt or 0.1g of sodium per 100g of food.

Ready-made foods are often higher in salt than the homemade equivalent, so this is another good reason to emphasise home-cooked dishes.

Some meat and yeast extracts, often used for flavour, are high in salt. Use them sparingly, or instead experiment with a range of different herbs and spices, many of which have strong and distinctive flavours, which means you can reduce the amount of salt you add to food.

*Get active and try to be a healthy weight*
Many people find that sticking to a low GI diet is an excellent and satisfying way to lose weight. The only guaranteed way to lose weight (and body fat) is to use up more energy (calories) than you consume, so the calorie counts provided in this book will help you to calculate how many you are taking in. Remember to aim at losing only 0.5–1kg per week .

Becoming more active by including activities like walking in daily life will burn up some of the calories, and is more likely to be sustained than a gym membership which involves travelling any distance.

*Drink plenty of water*
We all need over a litre of water each day as part of the recommended total intake of 2 litres of fluid. Water is calorie free and 0 GI, so it can be taken freely. All types of water are good for hydration and increasingly there is a trend away from bottled water towards fresh, chilled tap water.

Sugary drinks provide extra calories, as does alcohol, which can also be damaging to the liver if taken in excess.

Teas and coffees contain caffeine and while excessive amounts are harmful, normal quantities (3–4 cups a day) add to that all-important fluid intake. Try to use skimmed or semi-skimmed milk and avoid adding sugar. If you have a weakness for lattes, remember that many are made with full-fat milk to help the froth hold up.

*Don't skip breakfast*

This is one of the most important meals of the day, and is very easy to take in the form of a low GI food like porridge. Without breakfast our blood sugar can slump mid-morning, which makes us more likely to succumb to the temptation of a high calorie snack such as boiled sweets or sweet biscuits, which give an instant energy boost. It is no wonder that breakfast eaters tend to be slimmer! If you have to get up at the crack of dawn and rush for a train, then have something like fruit or a low GI cereal when you get to work.

### ALCOHOL

**The maximum amount of alcohol recommended each week for a woman is 21 units and for a man 28 units.**

**A unit is a pub measure of spirits, half a pint of beer, lager or cider and a small glass of wine.**

**Everyone is recommended to have at least one alcohol free day per week.**

### FINALLY

This GI counter aims to help you to eat a healthy low GI diet. Do not be obsessive about it, but use it for guidance and remember that there are no bad foods – but there are unbalanced and bad diets!

## A few reminders on using these tables

● Remember that 'low' GI foods are those with a GI below 55, 'medium' are those between 56 and 69 and 'high' those with a GI of 70 and above.

● GI may differ from brand to brand of the same food, so use these figures as a guide rather than absolute values.

● Information on the energy content of food is given in kcal per 100g.

● Carbohydrate content, fat and sodium levels are also per 100g.

● If you are a woman trying to lose weight, aim for 1500 kcal a day; if a man, 2000 kcal each day.

● A healthy diet includes less than 70g per day of fat if you are a woman and less than 95g if you are a man.

● Keep salt levels to less than 6g per day. Multiply the sodium figure given in these tables by 2.5 to convert to salt content.

# FRUITS
**including dried fruits, tinned fruits & juices**

We are all recommended to have five portions of fruit and vegetables each day. Try to vary the fruit you eat and not just stick to the same ones each day. And you don't have to eat a piece of fruit on its own: berry fruits have low GI levels and can be added to all sorts of dishes, like cereals and puddings.

Remember that nibbling on lots of dried fruit and slurping fruit juices can add extra calories.

|                                    | GI | kcal | Carbs g | Fat g | Sodium mg |
|------------------------------------|----|------|---------|-------|-----------|
| **Apple, average**                 | 38 | 47   | 10.5    | 0.1   | 3         |
| **Apple, Braeburn**                | 32 | 47   | 10.5    | 0.1   | 3         |
| **Apple, Golden Delicious**        | 39 | 47   | 10.5    | 0.1   | 3         |
| **Apple, baked, no sugar**         | 38 | 43   | 10.7    | 0.1   | 3         |
| **Apple, baked, with sugar**       | 38 | 78   | 20.1    | 0.1   | 3         |
| **Apple, dried**                   | 38 | 238  | 60.1    | 0.5   | 16        |
| **Apricots, fresh**                | 57 | 31   | 7.2     | 0.1   | 2         |
| **Apricots, tinned in juice**      | 64 | 34   | 8.4     | 0.1   | 5         |
| **Apricots, dried**                | 30 | 188  | 43.4    | 0.7   | 56        |
| **Avocado**                        | 1  | 190  | 1.9     | 19.3  | 6         |
| **Banana, average**                | 52 | 95   | 23.2    | 0.3   | 1         |
| **Banana, underripe**              | 42 | 95   | 23.2    | 0.3   | 1         |
| **Banana, overripe**               | 52 | 95   | 23.2    | 0.3   | 1         |
| **Blackberries**                   | 40 | 25   | 5.1     | 0.2   | 2         |
| **Cherries**                       | 22 | 48   | 11.5    | 0.1   | 1         |
| **Cherries, tinned in light syrup**| 22 | 71   | 18.5    | trace | 8         |
| **Cherry pie filling**             | 48 | 82   | 21.5    | trace | 30        |

|  | GI | kcal | Carbs g | Fat g | Sodium mg |
|---|---|---|---|---|---|
| **Cranberry juice** | 56 | 61 | 14.4 | 0 | no figure |
| **Cranberry juice drink** | 56 | 48 | 11.5 | 0.1 | 100 |
| **Currants** | 64 | 267 | 67.8 | 0.4 | 14 |
| **Dates, dried** | 103 | 270 | 68 | 0.2 | 10 |
| **Figs, dried** | 61 | 227 | 52.9 | 1.6 | 62 |
| **Figs, dried, cooked without sugar** | 61 | 126 | 29.4 | 0.9 | 34 |
| **Fruit cocktail, tinned in syrup** | 5 | 57 | 7.2 | trace | 3 |
| **Grapefruit** | 30 | 30 | 6.8 | 0.1 | 3 |
| **Grapes, black** | 59 | 60 | 15.4 | 0.1 | 2 |
| **Grapes, red** | 53 | 60 | 15.4 | 0.1 | 2 |
| **Grapes, white** | 53 | 60 | 15.4 | 0.1 | 2 |
| **Kiwi fruit** | 53 | 49 | 10.6 | 0.5 | 4 |
| **Kiwi fruit, Australia** | 58 | 49 | 10.6 | 0.5 | 4 |
| **Kiwi fruit, New Zealand** | 47 | 49 | 10.6 | 0.5 | 4 |
| **Lemon** | 42 | 19 | 3.2 | 0.3 | 5 |
| **Lychees in syrup, drained** | 79 | 68 | 17.7 | trace | 2 |
| **Mandarins, tinned in juice** | 42 | 32 | 7.7 | trace | 6 |

|  | GI | kcal | Carbs g | Fat g | Sodium mg |
|---|---|---|---|---|---|
| **Mandarins, tinned in syrup** | 42 | 52 | 13.4 | trace | 6 |
| **Mango** | 51 | 57 | 14.1 | 0.2 | 2 |
| **Melon, canteloupe** | 65 | 19 | 4.2 | 0.1 | 8 |
| **Melon, honeydew** | 65 | 28 | 6.6 | 0.1 | 32 |
| **Nectarines** | 42 | 40 | 9 | 0.1 | 1 |
| **Oranges** | 42 | 37 | 8.5 | 0.1 | 5 |
| **Papaya** | 56 | 45 | 11.3 | 0.1 | 4 |
| **Paw paw** | 56 | 36 | 8.8 | 0.1 | 5 |
| **Peaches, fresh** | 42 | 33 | 7.6 | 0.1 | 1 |
| **Peaches, tinned in heavy syrup** | 58 | 55 | 14 | trace | 4 |
| **Peaches, tinned in light syrup** | 57 | 55 | 14 | trace | 4 |
| **Peaches, tinned in juice** | 45 | 39 | 9.7 | trace | 12 |
| **Pears, fresh** | 38 | 40 | 10 | 0.1 | 3 |
| **Pears, tinned in juice** | 45 | 33 | 8.5 | trace | 3 |
| **Pineapple, fresh** | 66 | 41 | 10.1 | 0.2 | 2 |
| **Pineapple, tinned in juice** | 46 | 47 | 12.2 | trace | 1 |

| | GI | kcal | Carbs g | Fat g | Sodium mg |
|---|---|---|---|---|---|
| **Plums, fresh** | 24 | 36 | 8.8 | 0.1 | 2 |
| **Plums, tinned** | 39 | 59 | 15.5 | trace | 6 |
| **Prunes** | 29 | 141 | 38.4 | 0.5 | 12 |
| **Prunes, stewed, no sugar** | 29 | 81 | 19.5 | 0.3 | 6 |
| **Prunes, stewed, with sugar** | 29 | 103 | 25.5 | 0.2 | 5 |
| **Raisins** | 64 | 272 | 69.3 | 0.4 | 60 |
| **Raspberries** | 40 | 25 | 4.6 | 0.3 | 3 |
| **Rhubarb, raw** | 0 | 7 | 0.8 | 0.1 | 3 |
| **Rhubarb, stewed, no sugar** | 0 | 7 | 0.7 | 0.1 | 1 |
| **Strawberries** | 40 | 27 | 6 | 0.1 | 6 |
| **Sultanas** | 56 | 275 | 69.4 | 0.4 | 19 |
| **Tangerines** | 42 | 35 | 8 | 0.1 | 2 |
| **Watermelon, no skin** | 72 | 31 | 7.1 | 0.3 | 2 |

# VEGETABLES
**including dried, frozen & tinned**

In general these have a low GI and are part of the important five-a-day portions of fruit and vegetables that we should all eat. Try to vary them, and include large portions of vegetables or salads at lunch and evening meals as often as possible.

Even if you succumb to a ready-made meal accompany this with extra vegetables which can be cooked in a microwave for quickness. Obviously fresh vegetables are best, but frozen ones have the vitamins locked into them and even the tinned ones retain the fibre along with some vitamins.

Making vegetables into soups is a good way of eating them and one which children also often enjoy.

Between meals, try snacking on carrot sticks or raw celery rather than sweets.

|  | GI | kcal | Carbs g | Fat g | Sodium mg |
|---|---|---|---|---|---|
| **Alfalfa** | 1 | 24 | 0.4 | 0.7 | 6 |
| **Artichoke** | 1 | 18 | 2.7 | 0.2 | 27 |
| **Artichoke, tinned, average** | 0 | 30 | 5.5 | 0.1 | no figure |
| **Artichoke, globe, boiled, unsalted water** | 0 | 18 | 2.7 | 0.2 | 15 |
| **Artichoke, Jerusalem, boiled, unsalted water** | 0 | 41 | 10.6 | 0.1 | 3 |
| **Asparagus, raw** | 1 | 25 | 2 | 0.6 | 1 |
| **Asparagus, boiled** | 1 | 26 | 1.4 | 0.8 | 60 |
| **Aubergine, raw** | 1 | 15 | 2.2 | 0.4 | 2 |
| **Aubergine, fried** | 1 | 190 | 2.8 | 31.9 | 2 |
| **Avocado, raw** | 1 | 190 | 1.9 | 19.3 | 6 |
| **Bean sprouts, raw** | 1 | 31 | 4 | 0.5 | 5 |
| **Bean sprouts, stir-fried in oil** | 1 | 72 | 2.5 | 6.1 | 3 |
| **Beetroot** | 64 | 36 | 7.6 | 0.1 | 66 |
| **Broccoli, raw, green** | 1 | 33 | 1.8 | 0.9 | 8 |
| **Broccoli, boiled, green, unsalted water** | 1 | 24 | 1.1 | 0.8 | 13 |
| **Broccoli, boiled, green, salted water** | 1 | 24 | 1.1 | 0.8 | 150 |

| | GI | kcal | Carbs g | Fat g | Sodium mg |
|---|---|---|---|---|---|
| **Broccoli, purple-sprouting, raw** | 0 | 35 | 2.6 | 1.1 | 10 |
| **Broccoli, purple-sprouting, boiled, unsalted water** | 0 | 19 | 1.3 | 0.6 | 6 |
| **Broccoli, purple-sprouting, boiled, salted water** | 0 | 19 | 1.3 | 0.6 | 66 |
| **Brussels sprouts, raw** | 1 | 42 | 4.1 | 1.4 | 6 |
| **Brussels sprouts, boiled, unsalted water** | 1 | 35 | 3.5 | 1.3 | 2 |
| **Brussels sprouts, boiled, salted water** | 1 | 35 | 3.5 | 1.3 | 73 |
| **Cabbage, raw** | 1 | 26 | 4.1 | 0.4 | 5 |
| **Cabbage, boiled, unsalted water** | 1 | 16 | 2.2 | 0.4 | 8 |
| **Cabbage, boiled, salted water** | 1 | 16 | 2.2 | 0.4 | 120 |
| **Cabbage, Chinese, raw** | 0 | 12 | 1.4 | 0.2 | 7 |
| **Cabbage, average, dried** | 0 | 237 | 38 | 3.6 | 45 |
| **Cabbage, January King, raw** | 0 | 25 | 3.9 | 0.4 | 3 |
| **Cabbage, January King, boiled, salted water** | 0 | 18 | 2.5 | 0.6 | 100 |
| **Cabbage, red, raw** | 0 | 21 | 3.7 | 0.3 | 8 |

| | GI | kcal | Carbs g | Fat g | Sodium mg |
|---|---|---|---|---|---|
| **Cabbage, red, boiled salted water** | 0 | 15 | 2.3 | 0.3 | 130 |
| **Cabbage, Savoy, raw** | 0 | 27 | 3.9 | 0.5 | 5 |
| **Cabbage, Savoy, boiled, salted water** | 0 | 17 | 2.2 | 0.5 | 120 |
| **Cabbage, summer, raw** | 0 | 24 | 3.7 | 0.4 | 7 |
| **Cabbage, summer, boiled, salted water** | 0 | 14 | 1.8 | 0.4 | 140 |
| **Cabbage, white, raw** | 0 | 27 | 5 | 0.2 | 7 |
| **Cabbage, white, boiled, salted water** | 0 | 14 | 2.2 | 0.2 | 110 |
| **Carrots** | 49 | 35 | 7.9 | 0.3 | 25 |
| **Cassava, boiled** | 46 | 130 | 33.5 | 0.2 | 4 |
| **Cauliflower, raw** | 1 | 34 | 3 | 0.9 | 9 |
| **Cauliflower, boiled, unsalted water** | 0 | 28 | 2.1 | 0.9 | 4 |
| **Cauliflower, boiled, salted water** | 0 | 28 | 2.1 | 0.9 | 60 |
| **Celery, raw** | 0 | 7 | 0.9 | 0.2 | 60 |
| **Celery, boiled, salted water** | 0 | 8 | 0.8 | 0.3 | 160 |
| **Chard, Swiss, raw** | 0 | 19 | 2.9 | 0.2 | 210 |

| | GI | kcal | Carbs g | Fat g | Sodium mg |
|---|---|---|---|---|---|
| **Chard, Swiss, boiled, unsalted water** | 0 | 20 | 3.2 | 0.1 | 180 |
| **Chicory, raw** | 0 | 11 | 2.8 | 0.6 | 1 |
| **Chicory, boiled, salted water** | 0 | 7 | 2.1 | 0.3 | 150 |
| **Chillis** | 0 | 26 | 4.2 | 0.3 | 12 |
| **Chinese leaves** | 1 | 12 | 1.4 | 0.2 | no figure |
| **Courgette, raw** | 1 | 18 | 1.8 | 0.4 | 1 |
| **Courgette, boiled, unsalted water** | 1 | 19 | 2 | 0.4 | 1 |
| **Courgette, fried** | 1 | 62 | 2.6 | 4.8 | 1 |
| **Cucumber** | 1 | 10 | 1.5 | 0.1 | 3 |
| **Curly kale, raw** | 1 | 33 | 1.4 | 1.6 | 43 |
| **Curly kale, boiled, salted water** | 1 | 24 | 1 | 1.1 | 100 |
| **Endive, raw** | 0 | 13 | 1 | 0.6 | 10 |
| **Fennel, raw** | 1 | 12 | 1.8 | 0.2 | 11 |
| **Fennel, boiled, salted water** | 1 | 11 | 1.5 | 0.2 | 96 |
| **Garlic** | 1 | 98 | 16.2 | 0.6 | 4 |
| **Garlic purée** | 1 | 380 | 16.9 | 38.6 | 2740 |

| | GI | kcal | Carbs g | Fat g | Sodium mg |
|---|---|---|---|---|---|
| **Gourd, raw** | 1 | 11 | 0.8 | 0.2 | 1 |
| **Green beans, raw** | 1 | 24 | 3.2 | 0.5 | trace |
| **Green beans, boiled** | 1 | 25 | 4.7 | 0.1 | 8 |
| **Kohl rabi, raw** | 0 | 23 | 3.7 | 0.2 | 4 |
| **Kohl rabi, boiled, salted water** | 0 | 18 | 3.1 | 0.2 | 110 |
| **Leeks, raw** | 1 | 22 | 2.9 | 0.5 | 2 |
| **Leeks, boiled, unsalted water** | 1 | 22 | 2.6 | 0.7 | 6 |
| **Leeks, boiled, salted water** | 1 | 22 | 2.6 | 0.7 | 81 |
| **Lettuce** | 1 | 14 | 1.7 | 0.5 | 3 |
| **Lettuce, Butterhead** | 0 | 12 | 1.2 | 0.6 | 5 |
| **Lettuce, Cos** | 0 | 16 | 1.7 | 0.6 | 1 |
| **Lettuce, iceberg** | 1 | 13 | 1.9 | 0.3 | 2 |
| **Lettuce, Webbs** | 0 | 13 | 2 | 0.3 | 4 |
| **Mangetout, raw** | 1 | 32 | 4.2 | 0.2 | 2 |
| **Mangetout, boiled, salted water** | 1 | 26 | 3.3 | 0.1 | 42 |
| **Mangetout, stir-fried** | 1 | 71 | 3.5 | 4.8 | 2 |

|  | GI | kcal | Carbs g | Fat g | Sodium mg |
|---|---|---|---|---|---|
| **Marrow, raw** | 1 | 12 | 2.2 | 0.2 | 1 |
| **Marrow, boiled, unsalted water** | 1 | 9 | 1.6 | 0.2 | 1 |
| **Marrow, boiled, salted water** | 1 | 9 | 1.6 | 0.2 | 100 |
| **Mushrooms, raw** | 1 | 13 | 0.4 | 0.5 | 5 |
| **Mushrooms, fried** | 1 | 157 | 0.3 | 16.2 | 4 |
| **Mustard & cress** | 1 | 13 | 0.4 | 0.6 | 19 |
| **Okra, raw** | 1 | 31 | 13 | 1.0 | 8 |
| **Okra, boiled, unsalted water** | 1 | 28 | 2.7 | 0.7 | 5 |
| **Okra, fried** | 1 | 269 | 4.4 | 26.1 | 13 |
| **Onions, raw** | 0 | 36 | 7.9 | 0.2 | 3 |
| **Onions, baked** | 0 | 103 | 22.3 | 0.6 | 8 |
| **Onions, fried** | 0 | 164 | 14.1 | 11.2 | 4 |
| **Onions, pickled** | 0 | 24 | 4.9 | 0.2 | 450 |
| **Pak choi** | 0 | 11 | 1.4 | 0.2 | no figure |
| **Parsnips, raw** | 97 | 64 | 12.5 | 1.1 | 10 |
| **Parsnips, boiled, unsalted water** | 97 | 64 | 12.5 | 1.1 | 10 |

| | GI | kcal | Carbs g | Fat g | Sodium mg |
|---|---|---|---|---|---|
| **Parsnips, boiled, salted water** | 97 | 66 | 12.9 | 1.2 | 120 |
| **Peas, petit pois** | 40 | 83 | 11.3 | 1.5 | 1 |
| **Peas, marrowfat** | 39 | 80 | 13 | 0.4 | 0 |
| **Pepper, chilli** | 1 | 20 | 0.7 | 0.6 | 7 |
| **Peppers, green, raw** | 1 | 15 | 2.6 | 0.3 | 4 |
| **Peppers, green boiled, salted water** | 1 | 18 | 2.6 | 0.5 | 70 |
| **Peppers, red, raw** | 1 | 32 | 6.4 | 0.4 | 4 |
| **Peppers, red, boiled, salted water** | 1 | 34 | 7 | 0.4 | 70 |
| **Pumpkin, raw** | 75 | 13 | 2.2 | 0.2 | trace |
| **Pumpkin, boiled, salted water** | 75 | 13 | 2.1 | 0.3 | 76 |
| **Raddicchio** | 0 | 14 | 1.7 | 0.2 | 7 |
| **Radishes** | 1 | 12 | 1.9 | 0.2 | 11 |
| **Salad leaves** | 1 | 17 | 2 | 0.2 | trace |
| **Sauerkraut** | 0 | 9 | 1.1 | trace | 590 |
| **Shallots, raw** | 0 | 20 | 3.3 | 0.2 | 10 |
| **Shallots, pickled** | 0 | 77 | 18 | 0.1 | no figure |

|  | GI | kcal | Carbs g | Fat g | Sodium mg |
|---|---|---|---|---|---|
| **Spinach, raw** | 1 | 25 | 1.6 | 0.8 | 140 |
| **Spinach, boiled, unsalted water** | 1 | 19 | 0.8 | 0.8 | 120 |
| **Spinach, boiled, salted water** | 1 | 19 | 0.8 | 0.8 | 210 |
| **Spring greens, raw** | 1 | 33 | 31 | 1.0 | 20 |
| **Spring greens, boiled, unsalted water** | 1 | 20 | 1.6 | 0.7 | 10 |
| **Spring greens, boiled, salted water** | 1 | 20 | 1.6 | 0.7 | 79 |
| **Swede** | 72 | 24 | 5 | 0.3 | 15 |
| **Sweetcorn, drained, baby, tinned** | 46 | 23 | 2 | 0.4 | 1140 |
| **Sweetcorn on cob, boiled, unsalted water** | 48 | 66 | 11.6 | 1.4 | 1 |
| **Sweetcorn on cob, boiled, salted water** | 48 | 66 | 11.6 | 1.4 | 9 |
| **Watercress** | 1 | 22 | 0.4 | 1.0 | 49 |
| **Yam, boiled, unsalted water** | 37 | 133 | 33 | 0.3 | 17 |
| **Yam, boiled, salted water** | 37 | 133 | 33 | 0.3 | 72 |

# POTATOES

Potatoes make a useful substantial accompaniment to a meal but, with the exception of sweet potatoes, they have a relatively high GI. Small potatoes boiled in their skins have lower GI levels than average and also contain more fibre as the skins are eaten.

Obviously crisps and French fries have a low GI because the fat content reduces the overall GI – but if you overindulge the fat and calories become a problem. Low-fat oven chips are a healthy choice – or, better still, make your own from thick-cut potato chips, brush them with oil and then oven bake them. They can be made from sweet potatoes for an unusual flavour.

| | GI | kcal | Carbs g | Fat g | Sodium mg |
|---|---|---|---|---|---|
| **Potatoes, baked** | 85 | 136 | 31.7 | 0.2 | 12 |
| **Potatoes, crisp** | 57 | 530 | 53.3 | 34.2 | 800 |
| **Potatoes, Desirée, boiled** | 101 | 74 | 17 | 0.2 | 8 |
| **Potatoes, French fries, microwaved** | 75 | 221 | 32.1 | 10.2 | 40 |
| **Potatoes, mashed** | 74 | 72 | 17.0 | 0.1 | 7 |
| **Potatoes, mashed, instant** | 86 | 57 | 13.5 | 0.1 | 200 |
| **Potatoes, new, tinned, reheated, drained** | 65 | 66 | 15.1 | 0.1 | 250 |
| **Potatoes, new, unpeeled, boiled in skins** | 76 | 75 | 17.8 | 0.3 | 9 |
| **Potatoes, peeled and boiled** | 101 | 72 | 17.0 | 0.1 | 7 |
| **Potatoes, sweet, boiled** | 46 | 84 | 20.5 | 0.3 | 32 |

# FISH, SHELLFISH & SEAFOOD

Fish, shellfish and sea foods such as seaweed all have a GI of 0 and are a good source of protein and minerals. Oily fish is also a good source of omega-3 fatty acids (see page 14).

|  | GI | kcal | Carbs g | Fat g | Sodium mg |
|---|---|---|---|---|---|
| **Anchovies, tinned in oil** | 0 | 191 | 0 | 10 | 3930 |
| **Bass, raw** | 0 | 100 | 0 | 2.5 | 69 |
| **Bream, raw** | 0 | 96 | 0 | 2.9 | 110 |
| **Catfish, raw** | 0 | 96 | 0 | 2.8 | 95 |
| **Catfish, steamed** | 0 | 119 | 0 | 3.7 | 110 |
| **Clams in brine** | 0 | 77 | 1.9 | 0.6 | 1200 |
| **Cockles, boiled** | 0 | 53 | 0 | 0.6 | 490 |
| **Cod fillet, raw** | 0 | 80 | 0 | 0.7 | 60 |
| **Cod fillet, baked** | 0 | 96 | trace | 1.2 | 340 |
| **Cod fillet, grilled** | 0 | 80 | trace | 1.3 | 91 |
| **Cod fillet, poached** | 0 | 94 | trace | 1.1 | 110 |
| **Cod, smoked, raw** | 0 | 79 | 0 | 0.6 | 1170 |
| **Cod, smoked, poached** | 0 | 101 | trace | 1.6 | 1200 |
| **Cod, steamed** | 0 | 83 | 0 | 0.9 | 65 |
| **Cod, dried & salted, raw** | 0 | 130 | 0 | 0.7 | no figure |
| **Cod, dried & salted, boiled** | 0 | 138 | 0 | 0.9 | 400 |
| **Coley, raw** | 0 | 82 | 0 | 1.0 | 86 |
| **Coley, steamed** | 0 | 82 | 0 | 1.3 | 97 |

| | GI | kcal | Carbs g | Fat g | Sodium mg |
|---|---|---|---|---|---|
| **Crab meat, boiled** | 0 | 128 | 0 | 5.5 | 420 |
| **Crab, tinned in brine** | 0 | 77 | 0 | 0.5 | 550 |
| **Dab, raw** | 0 | 74 | 0 | 1.2 | 77 |
| **Eel, raw** | 0 | 168 | 0 | 11.3 | 89 |
| **Eels, jellied** | 0 | 98 | trace | 7.1 | 660 |
| **Fish fingers, oven-baked** | 38 | 200 | 16.6 | 8.9 | 440 |
| **Fish fingers, raw** | 38 | 171 | 14.2 | 7.8 | 470 |
| **Haddock, raw** | 0 | 81 | 0 | 0.6 | 67 |
| **Haddock, grilled** | 0 | 104 | 0 | 0.8 | 86 |
| **Haddock, steamed** | 0 | 89 | 0 | 0.6 | 73 |
| **Haddock, smoked, raw** | 0 | 81 | 0 | 0.6 | 760 |
| **Haddock, smoked, steamed** | 0 | 101 | 0 | 0.9 | 990 |
| **Hake, raw** | 0 | 92 | 0 | 2.2 | 100 |
| **Hake, grilled** | 0 | 113 | 0 | 2.7 | 130 |
| **Halibut, raw** | 0 | 103 | 0 | 1.9 | 60 |
| **Halibut, grilled** | 0 | 121 | 0 | 2.2 | 71 |
| **Halibut, steamed** | 0 | 131 | 0 | 4.0 | 110 |
| **Herring, raw** | 0 | 190 | 0 | 13.2 | 120 |

| | GI | kcal | Carbs g | Fat g | Sodium mg |
|---|---|---|---|---|---|
| **Herring, dried & salted** | 0 | 168 | 0 | 7.4 | 520 |
| **Herring, fried** | 0 | 234 | 1.5 | 15.1 | 100 |
| **Herring, grilled** | 0 | 181 | 0 | 11.2 | 160 |
| **Herring, pickled** | 0 | 209 | 10 | 11.1 | 830 |
| **Hoki, raw** | 0 | 85 | 0 | 1.9 | 86 |
| **Hoki, grilled** | 0 | 121 | 0 | 2.7 | 120 |
| **Kippers, raw** | 0 | 229 | 0 | 17.7 | 830 |
| **Kippers, baked** | 0 | 205 | 0 | 11.4 | 990 |
| **Kippers, grilled** | 0 | 161 | 0 | 12.2 | 590 |
| **Lemon sole, raw** | 0 | 83 | 0 | 1.5 | 95 |
| **Lemon sole, grilled** | 0 | 97 | 0 | 1.7 | 110 |
| **Lemon sole, steamed** | 0 | 91 | 0 | 0.9 | 120 |
| **Lobster, boiled** | 0 | 103 | 0 | 1.6 | 330 |
| **Mackerel, raw** | 0 | 220 | 0 | 16.1 | 63 |
| **Mackerel, fried** | 0 | 272 | 0 | 19.5 | 81 |
| **Mackerel, grilled** | 0 | 239 | 0 | 17.3 | 63 |
| **Mackerel in brine** | 0 | 237 | 0 | 17.9 | 270 |
| **Mackerel in olive oil** | 0 | 298 | 1 | 24.4 | no figure |

|  | GI | kcal | Carbs g | Fat g | Sodium mg |
|---|---|---|---|---|---|
| **Mackerel, peppered** | 0 | 310 | 0.3 | 25.2 | no figure |
| **Mackerel, smoked** | 0 | 354 | 0 | 30.9 | 750 |
| **Marlin, raw** | 0 | 99 | 0 | 0.2 | no figure |
| **Marlin, chargrilled** | 0 | 153 | 0.8 | 6.1 | no figure |
| **Marlin, smoked** | 0 | 120 | 0 | 0.1 | no figure |
| **Monkfish, raw** | 0 | 66 | 0 | 0.4 | 18 |
| **Monkfish, grilled** | 0 | 96 | 0 | 0.6 | 26 |
| **Mullet, grey, raw** | 0 | 115 | 0 | 4 | 65 |
| **Mullet, grey, grilled** | 0 | 150 | 0 | 5.2 | 84 |
| **Mullet, red, raw** | 0 | 109 | 0 | 3.8 | 91 |
| **Mullet, red, grilled** | 0 | 121 | 0 | 4.4 | 110 |
| **Mussels, raw** | 0 | 74 | 2.5 | 2.8 | 290 |
| **Mussels, boiled, no shell** | 0 | 28 | 3.5 | 2.7 | 360 |
| **Mussels, boiled, with shells** | 0 | 28 | 0.9 | 0.7 | 96 |
| **Octopus, raw** | 0 | 83 | trace | 1.3 | no figure |
| **Oysters** | 0 | 65 | 2.7 | 1.3 | 510 |
| **Pilchards in tomato sauce** | 0 | 144 | 1.1 | 8.1 | 290 |
| **Pilchards in brine** | 0 | 148 | 0 | 7.3 | no figure |

| | GI | kcal | Carbs g | Fat g | Sodium mg |
|---|---|---|---|---|---|
| **Plaice, raw** | 0 | 79 | 0 | 1.4 | 120 |
| **Plaice, grilled** | 0 | 96 | 0 | 1.7 | 140 |
| **Plaice, steamed** | 0 | 93 | 0 | 1.9 | 120 |
| **Prawns, raw** | 0 | 76 | 0 | 0.6 | 190 |
| **Prawns, peeled, boiled in salt water** | 0 | 99 | 0 | 0.9 | 1590 |
| **Rock salmon/dogfish, raw** | 0 | 154 | 0 | 9.7 | 120 |
| **Roe, cod's** | 0 | 104 | 0 | 1.9 | 110 |
| **Salmon, fresh** | 0 | 180 | 0 | 11.0 | 45 |
| **Salmon, grilled** | 0 | 215 | 0 | 13.1 | 54 |
| **Salmon, pink, tinned in brine** | 0 | 153 | 0 | 7.8 | 430 |
| **Salmon, smoked** | 0 | 142 | 0 | 4.5 | 1880 |
| **Salmon, steamed** | 0 | 194 | 0 | 11.9 | 49 |
| **Sardines, fresh** | 0 | 165 | 0 | 9.2 | 120 |
| **Sardines, tinned in brine** | 0 | 172 | 0 | 9.5 | 530 |
| **Sardines, tinned in oil** | 0 | 220 | 0 | 14.1 | 450 |
| **Sardines, grilled** | 0 | 195 | 0 | 10.4 | 140 |

| | GI | kcal | Carbs g | Fat g | Sodium mg |
|---|---|---|---|---|---|
| **Sardines, in tomato sauce** | 0 | 162 | 1.4 | 9.9 | 350 |
| **Scallops, steamed** | 0 | 118 | 3.4 | 1.1 | 18 |
| **Seaweed, Irish moss, dried, raw** | 0 | 8 | trace | 0.2 | 67 |
| **Seaweed, kombu, dried, raw** | 0 | 43 | trace | 1.6 | 1830 |
| **Seaweed nori, dried, raw** | 0 | 136 | trace | 1.5 | 790 |
| **Seaweed, wakame, dried, raw** | 0 | 71 | trace | 2.4 | 3220 |
| **Shark, raw** | 0 | 102 | 0 | 1.1 | 140 |
| **Shrimps, boiled** | 0 | 117 | trace | 2.4 | 3840 |
| **Shrimps, tinned in brine** | 0 | 94 | 0 | 1.2 | 980 |
| **Shrimps, frozen** | 0 | 73 | 0 | 0.8 | 380 |
| **Skate, raw** | 0 | 64 | 0 | 0.4 | 120 |
| **Skate, grilled** | 0 | 79 | 0 | 0.5 | 150 |
| **Snapper, red, raw** | 0 | 90 | 0 | 1.3 | 77 |
| **Snapper, red, fried** | 0 | 126 | 0 | 3.1 | 120 |
| **Squid** | 0 | 70 | 1.2 | 1.7 | 110 |
| **Sushi** | 0 | 143 | 24.3 | 2.2 | 400 |
| **Swordfish, raw** | 0 | 109 | 0 | 4.1 | 130 |

| | GI | kcal | Carbs g | Fat g | Sodium mg |
|---|---|---|---|---|---|
| **Swordfish, grilled** | 0 | 139 | 0 | 5.2 | 170 |
| **Trout fillet, raw** | 0 | 125 | 0 | 5.2 | 45 |
| **Trout fillet, grilled** | 0 | 135 | 0 | 5.4 | 55 |
| **Trout fillet steamed** | 0 | 135 | 0 | 4.5 | 88 |
| **Trout, brown, raw** | 0 | 112 | 0 | 3.8 | 56 |
| **Trout, smoked** | 0 | 139 | 0.3 | 5.2 | no figure |
| **Tuna, fresh** | 0 | 136 | 0 | 4.6 | 47 |
| **Tuna in spring water** | 0 | 108 | 0 | 0.6 | no figure |
| **Tuna, tinned in brine** | 0 | 99 | 0 | 0.6 | 320 |
| **Tuna, tinned in oil** | 0 | 189 | 0 | 9.0 | 290 |
| **Tuna, tinned in water** | 0 | 105 | 0.1 | 0.8 | no figure |
| **Tuna pâté** | 0 | 236 | 0.4 | 18.6 | 390 |
| **Turbot, raw** | 0 | 95 | 0 | 2.7 | 68 |
| **Turbot, grilled** | 0 | 122 | 0 | 3.5 | 9 |
| **Whitebait, fried in flour** | 0 | 525 | 5.3 | 47.5 | 230 |
| **Whelks, boiled** | 0 | 89 | trace | 1.2 | 280 |
| **Whiting, raw** | 0 | 81 | 0 | 0.7 | 90 |
| **Whiting, steamed** | 0 | 92 | 0 | 0.9 | 110 |
| **Winkles** | 0 | 72 | trace | 1.2 | 750 |

# RED MEAT

Fresh meat has a GI of 0. But when carbohydrate is added – such as rusk in sausages – this produces a higher GI. Choose lean meat to reduce the fat content. Vary the types of meat you use and experiment with different cuts.

Red meat such as beef, lamb and pork provides iron in an easily absorbed form. We all need iron, especially women due to the monthly blood loss. Liver is another good source of iron and if you use small, thin slices in dishes like stir fries and casseroles you may persuade children to try it! Also liver can be easily made into pâtés. As liver has a high level of vitamin A it is not recommended for pregnant women.

Combining meat with pulses in dishes such as casseroles and curries really keeps the fat content down and the GI level low.

|                                            | GI | kcal | Carbs g | Fat g | Sodium mg |
|--------------------------------------------|----|------|---------|-------|-----------|
| Bacon, back rasher, raw                    | 0  | 136  | 0       | 6.7   | 1350      |
| Bacon, back rasher, grilled                | 0  | 287  | 0       | 21.6  | 1880      |
| Bacon, back rasher, microwaved             | 0  | 307  | 0       | 23.3  | 2330      |
| Bacon, back rasher, reduced salt, grilled  | 0  | 282  | 0       | 20.6  | 1130      |
| Bacon back, crispy, grilled                | 0  | 313  | 0       | 18.8  | 2700      |
| Bacon back, dry fried                      | 0  | 295  | 0       | 22    | 1910      |
| Bacon, back, fat trimmed, raw              | 0  | 136  | 0       | 6.7   | 1350      |
| Bacon, back, fat trimmed, grilled          | 0  | 214  | 0       | 12.3  | 1930      |
| Bacon back, smoked, grilled                | 0  | 293  | 0       | 22.1  | 1760      |
| Bacon back, sweetcure, grilled             | 0  | 258  | 1.6     | 17.4  | 1790      |
| Bacon back, tendersure, grilled            | 0  | 213  | trace   | 11.9  | 1990      |
| Bacon, middle, raw                         | 0  | 241  | 0       | 20    | 1480      |
| Bacon, middle, fried                       | 0  | 350  | 0       | 28.5  | 1840      |
| Bacon, middle, grilled                     | 0  | 307  | 0       | 23.1  | 1960      |

|  | GI | kcal | Carbs g | Fat g | Sodium mg |
|---|---|---|---|---|---|
| **Bacon streaky fried** | 0 | 335 | 0 | 26.6 | 1880 |
| **Bacon, streaky rasher, raw** | 0 | 276 | 0 | 23.6 | 1260 |
| **Bacon, streaky rasher, grilled** | 0 | 337 | 0 | 26.9 | 1680 |
| **Bacon, loin steaks, grilled** | 0 | 191 | 0 | 9.7 | 1480 |
| **Bacon, collar joint, raw** | 0 | 319 | 0 | 28.9 | 1690 |
| **Bacon, collar joint, boiled** | 0 | 325 | 0 | 27 | 1100 |
| **Bacon, gammon joint, raw** | 0 | 138 | 0 | 7.5 | 880 |
| **Bacon, gammon joint, boiled** | 0 | 204 | 0 | 12.7 | 1180 |
| **Beef, braising steak, raw** | 0 | 225 | 0 | 9.7 | 62 |
| **Beef, braising steak, slow cooked** | 0 | 197 | 0 | 7.9 | 53 |
| **Beef braising steak lean raw** | 0 | 139 | 0 | 5.7 | 64 |
| **Beef, braising steak, lean, slow-cooked** | 0 | 197 | 0 | 7.9 | 53 |
| **Beef, braising steak, lean, braised** | 0 | 225 | 0 | 9.7 | 62 |
| **Beef, braising steak, lean & fat, raw** | 0 | 160 | 0 | 8.6 | 60 |

| | GI | kcal | Carbs g | Fat g | Sodium mg |
|---|---|---|---|---|---|
| **Beef, braising steak, lean & fat, slow-cooked** | 0 | 217 | 0 | 11.2 | 50 |
| **Beef, braising steak, lean & fat, braised** | 0 | 246 | 0 | 12.7 | 60 |
| **Beef, brisket, lean, raw** | 0 | 139 | 0 | 6.1 | 59 |
| **Beef, brisket, lean, boiled** | 0 | 225 | 0 | 11 | 50 |
| **Beef, brisket, lean & fat, raw** | 0 | 218 | 0 | 16 | 50 |
| **Beef, brisket, lean & fat, boiled** | 0 | 268 | 0 | 17.4 | 46 |
| **Beef flank, lean, raw** | 0 | 175 | 0 | 9.3 | 64 |
| **Beef flank, lean, pot roast** | 0 | 253 | 0 | 14 | 51 |
| **Beef flank, lean & fat, raw** | 0 | 266 | 0 | 20.8 | 54 |
| **Beef flank, lean & fat pot roast** | 0 | 309 | 0 | 22.3 | 45 |
| **Beef, fore-rib, lean, raw** | 0 | 145 | 0 | 6.5 | 61 |
| **Beef, fore-rib, lean, microwaved** | 0 | 243 | 0 | 11.4 | 60 |
| **Beef, fore-rib, lean, roast** | 0 | 236 | 0 | 11.4 | 57 |
| **Beef fore-rib, lean & fat, raw** | 0 | 253 | 0 | 19.8 | 52 |
| **Beef fore-rib, lean & fat, microwaved** | 0 | 300 | 0 | 20.4 | 54 |

|  | GI | kcal | Carbs g | Fat g | Sodium mg |
|---|---|---|---|---|---|
| **Beef, fore-rib, lean & fat, roast** | 0 | 306 | 0 | 20.5 | 54 |
| **Beef grillsteaks, raw** | 0 | 285 | 0.2 | 22.2 | 570 |
| **Beef grillsteaks, fried** | 0 | 302 | 0.5 | 22.2 | 800 |
| **Beef grillsteaks, grilled** | 0 | 305 | 0.5 | 23.9 | 710 |
| **Beef, lean, raw** | 0 | 132 | 0 | 5.1 | 64 |
| **Beef mince, raw** | 0 | 225 | 0 | 16.2 | 1080 |
| **Beef mince, stewed** | 0 | 209 | 0 | 13.5 | 73 |
| **Beef mince, microwaved** | 0 | 263 | 0 | 17.5 | 91 |
| **Beef mince, extra lean, raw** | 0 | 174 | 0 | 9.6 | 90 |
| **Beef mince, extra lean, stewed** | 0 | 177 | 0 | 8.7 | 75 |
| **Beef, rump steak, raw, lean & fat** | 0 | 174 | 0 | 10.1 | 56 |
| **Beef, rump steak, fried, lean** | 0 | 183 | 0 | 6.6 | 78 |
| **Beef, rump steak, grilled, lean** | 0 | 177 | 0 | 5.9 | 74 |
| **Beef, salted, raw** | 0 | 119 | 0 | 0.4 | no figure |
| **Beef, salted, raw, dried** | 0 | 250 | 0 | 1.5 | no figure |

| | GI | kcal | Carbs g | Fat g | Sodium mg |
|---|---|---|---|---|---|
| **Beef, silverside, lean, raw** | 0 | 134 | 0 | 4.3 | 62 |
| **Beef, silverside, lean, pot roast** | 0 | 193 | 0 | 6.3 | 58 |
| **Beef, silverside, lean, salted, boiled** | 0 | 184 | 0 | 6.9 | 1020 |
| **Beef sirloin, raw** | 0 | 201 | 0 | 12.7 | 62 |
| **Beef, sirloin, lean, raw** | 0 | 135 | 0 | 4.5 | 70 |
| **Beef, sirloin, lean, roast** | 0 | 188 | 0 | 6.5 | 55 |
| **Beef sirloin lean & fat, roast** | 0 | 233 | 0 | 12.6 | 53 |
| **Beef, stewing steak** | 0 | 146 | 0 | 6.4 | 66 |
| **Beef stewing steak, lean, raw** | 0 | 122 | 0 | 3.5 | 69 |
| **Beef stewing steak, lean, pressure cooked** | 0 | 199 | 0 | 6.5 | 60 |
| **Beef stewing steak, lean stewed** | 0 | 185 | 0 | 6.3 | 54 |
| **Beef topside, raw, lean & fat** | 0 | 198 | 0 | 12.9 | 67 |
| **Beef topside, medium rare** | 0 | 222 | 0 | 11.4 | 62 |
| **Beef topside, well done** | 0 | 244 | 0 | 12.5 | 57 |

| | GI | kcal | Carbs g | Fat g | Sodium mg |
|---|---|---|---|---|---|
| **Beef burgers, 99% meat, raw** | 0 | 291 | 0.1 | 24.7 | 290 |
| **Beef burgers, 99% meat, fried** | 0 | 329 | 0.1 | 23.9 | 470 |
| **Beef burgers, 99% meat, grilled** | 0 | 326 | 0.1 | 24.4 | 400 |
| **Beef, corned, tinned** | 0 | 205 | 1 | 10.9 | 860 |
| **Beef pie** | 45 | 299 | 22.1 | 19.4 | 460 |
| **Gammon steak, fat removed** | 0 | 138 | 0 | 7.5 | 880 |
| **Ham** | 0 | 107 | 1 | 3.3 | 1200 |
| **Heart, lamb's, raw** | 0 | 119 | 0 | 6.8 | 140 |
| **Heart, lamb's, roasted** | 0 | 226 | 0 | 13.9 | 84 |
| **Kidney, lamb's, fried** | 0 | 188 | 0 | 4.6 | 230 |
| **Kidney, ox, stewed** | 0 | 138 | 0 | 4.4 | 150 |
| **Kidney, pig's, stewed fried** | 0 | 153 | 0 | 6.1 | 370 |
| **Lamb, best end cutlets, lean, grilled** | 0 | 238 | 0 | 13.8 | 84 |
| **Lamb, best end cutlets, lean, barbecued** | 0 | 236 | 0 | 13.9 | 82 |
| **Lamb, best end cutlets lean & fat, grilled** | 0 | 367 | 0 | 29.9 | 81 |

| | GI | kcal | Carbs g | Fat g | Sodium mg |
|---|---|---|---|---|---|
| **Lamb, best end cutlets, lean & fat, barbecued** | 0 | 342 | 0 | 27.2 | 80 |
| **Lamb breast, lean, raw** | 0 | 179 | 0 | 11.2 | 86 |
| **Lamb breast, lean, roast** | 0 | 273 | 0 | 18.5 | 93 |
| **Lamb breast lean & fat, raw** | 0 | 287 | 0 | 24.7 | 69 |
| **Lamb breast, lean & fat, roast** | 0 | 359 | 0 | 29.9 | 85 |
| **Lamb chop with fat** | 0 | 277 | 0 | 23.0 | 63 |
| **Lamb kebab, grilled** | 0 | 288 | 0 | 19.3 | 87 |
| **Lamb, lean, raw** | 0 | 153 | 0 | 8.0 | 70 |
| **Lamb, leg, lean, roast** | 0 | 203 | 0 | 9.4 | 63 |
| **Lamb, leg, lean, braised** | 0 | 204 | 0 | 10.5 | 58 |
| **Lamb, loin chop, grilled, lean** | 0 | 213 | 0 | 10.7 | 80 |
| **Lamb, loin chop, grilled, with fat** | 0 | 277 | 0 | 22.1 | 81 |
| **Lamb mince, raw** | 0 | 196 | 0 | 13.3 | 69 |
| **Lamb mince, stewed** | 0 | 208 | 0 | 12.3 | 59 |
| **Lamb, neck fillet, raw** | 0 | 203 | 0 | 13.9 | 61 |
| **Lamb, neck fillet, grilled** | 0 | 284 | 0 | 19.1 | 78 |

|  | GI | kcal | Carbs g | Fat g | Sodium mg |
|---|---|---|---|---|---|
| **Lamb, shoulder, lean roast** | 0 | 235 | 0 | 13.5 | 75 |
| **Lamb, stewing, stewed** | 0 | 240 | 0 | 14.8 | 49 |
| **Liver, calf's, fried** | 0 | 188 | 0 | 9.6 | 70 |
| **Liver, chicken, fried** | 0 | 169 | 0 | 8.9 | 79 |
| **Liver, lamb's, fried** | 0 | 237 | 0 | 12.9 | 82 |
| **Liver, ox, stewed** | 0 | 198 | 3.6 | 9.5 | 110 |
| **Liver, pig's, stewed** | 0 | 189 | 3.6 | 8.1 | 130 |
| **Liver pâté** | 0 | 348 | 0.8 | 32.7 | 750 |
| **Liver pâté, reduced fat** | 0 | 191 | 3 | 12 | 710 |
| **Pork belly, grilled** | 0 | 320 | 0 | 23.4 | 97 |
| **Pork chop, lean & fat, raw** | 0 | 257 | 0 | 18.2 | 45 |
| **Pork chop, lean & fat, roasted** | 0 | 301 | 0 | 19.3 | 68 |
| **Pork diced, lean, raw** | 0 | 122 | 0 | 4 | 70 |
| **Pork, diced, lean, slow-cooked** | 0 | 169 | 0 | 5.4 | 41 |
| **Pork, diced, lean, casseroled** | 0 | 184 | 0 | 6.4 | 37 |
| **Pork diced, lean & fat, raw** | 0 | 147 | 0 | 7.2 | 68 |

|  | GI | kcal | Carbs g | Fat g | Sodium mg |
|---|---|---|---|---|---|
| **Pork diced, lean & fat, slow-cooked** | 0 | 173 | 0 | 6 | 42 |
| **Pork diced, lean, casseroled** | 0 | 184 | 0 | 6.8 | 37 |
| **Pork diced, kebabs, lean, grilled** | 0 | 179 | 0 | 4.7 | 80 |
| **Pork, diced, kebabs lean & fat, grilled** | 0 | 189 | 0 | 6.1 | 81 |
| **Pork fillet strips, stir-fried** | 0 | 182 | 0 | 5.9 | 71 |
| **Pork leg, raw, lean & fat** | 0 | 213 | 0 | 15.2 | 60 |
| **Pork leg, roasted, lean** | 0 | 182 | 0 | 5.5 | 69 |
| **Pork loin chop, raw, lean & fat** | 0 | 270 | 0 | 21.7 | 53 |
| **Pork loin chop, grilled, lean** | 0 | 184 | 0 | 6.4 | 66 |
| **Pork meat only, raw** | 0 | 128 | 0 | 4.0 | 70 |
| **Pork steak, raw, lean & fat** | 0 | 169 | 0 | 9.4 | 58 |
| **Pork steak, grilled, lean & fat** | 0 | 198 | 0 | 7.6 | 76 |
| **Salami** | 0 | 438 | 0.5 | 39.2 | 1800 |
| **Sausages, pork, fried** | 28 | 308 | 9.9 | 23.9 | 1070 |

| | GI | kcal | Carbs g | Fat g | Sodium mg |
|---|---|---|---|---|---|
| **Sausages, pork, grilled** | 28 | 294 | 9.8 | 22.1 | 1080 |
| **Shish kebab, meat** | 0 | 206 | 0 | 10 | 510 |
| **Tongue** | 0 | 201 | trace | 14.0 | 1000 |
| **Tripe raw** | 0 | 33 | 0 | 2.5 | 50 |
| **Tripe stewed** | 0 | 100 | 0 | 4.5 | 73 |
| **Veal, raw** | 0 | 109 | 0 | 2.7 | 110 |
| **Veal, roasted** | 0 | 230 | 0 | 11.5 | 97 |
| **Veal escalope, raw** | 0 | 106 | 0 | 1.7 | 59 |
| **Veal escalope, fried** | 0 | 196 | 0 | 6.8 | 86 |
| **Venison, raw** | 0 | 103 | 0 | 2.2 | 55 |
| **Venison, roasted** | 0 | 165 | 0 | 2.5 | 52 |

# POULTRY & GAME

These all have a GI of 0. They make a good contribution to protein in the diet. Try to vary them and remember to strip off the skin before eating.

Game like rabbit and pheasant makes a tasty and low-fat alternative to both chicken and turkey.

| | GI | kcal | Carbs g | Fat g | Sodium mg |
|---|---|---|---|---|---|
| **Chicken, leg quarter, meat & skin, raw** | 0 | 193 | 0 | 13.3 | 80 |
| **Chicken, leg quarter, meat & skin, casseroled** | 0 | 217 | 0 | 13.9 | 70 |
| **Chicken, leg quarter, meat & skin roast** | 0 | 236 | 0 | 16.9 | 95 |
| **Chicken, leg quarter, meat only, casseroled** | 0 | 176 | 0 | 8.4 | 75 |
| **Chicken, wing quarter, meat & skin, raw** | 0 | 193 | 0 | 12.4 | 60 |
| **Chicken, wing quarter, meat & skin, casseroled** | 0 | 210 | 0 | 12.5 | 60 |
| **Chicken, wing quarter, meat & skin, roast** | 0 | 226 | 0 | 14.1 | 100 |
| **Chicken, wing quarter, meat only, casseroled** | 0 | 164 | 0 | 6.3 | 65 |
| **Duck, meat only, raw** | 0 | 137 | 0 | 6.5 | 110 |
| **Duck, meat & skin, roasted** | 0 | 388 | 0 | 49.6 | 87 |
| **Duck, meat only, roasted** | 0 | 195 | 0 | 10.4 | 96 |
| **Duck, crispy Chinese** | 0 | 331 | 0.3 | 24.2 | 453 |
| **Goose, roasted, meat & skin** | 0 | 301 | 0 | 21.2 | 80 |

| | GI | kcal | Carbs g | Fat g | Sodium mg |
|---|---|---|---|---|---|
| **Pheasant, roasted, meat only** | 0 | 220 | 0 | 3.2 | 66 |
| **Poussin, raw** | 0 | 202 | 0 | 13.9 | 70 |
| **Rabbit, raw** | 0 | 137 | 0 | 5.5 | 67 |
| **Rabbit, stewed** | 0 | 114 | 0 | 3.4 | 48 |
| **Turkey, raw, dark meat only** | 0 | 105 | 0 | 2.5 | 90 |
| **Turkey, raw, light meat only** | 0 | 104 | 0 | 0.8 | 50 |
| **Turkey breast, grilled** | 0 | 155 | 0 | 1.7 | 90 |
| **Turkey, roast, meat & skin** | 0 | 171 | 0 | 6.5 | 52 |
| **Turkey strips, stir-fried** | 0 | 164 | 0 | 4.5 | 60 |

# EGGS

Eggs have a GI of 0 and are a good source of protein. They are convenient to make into a range of quick and easy dishes. As a change from omelettes, try them in savoury custards combined with vegetables.

Remember that egg yolks contain cholesterol, so if you are concerned about cholesterol levels you may be advised to limit your egg intake.

|                    | GI | kcal | Carbs g | Fat g | Sodium mg |
|--------------------|----|------|---------|-------|-----------|
| **Egg, boiled**        | 0  | 147  | trace   | 10.8  | 140       |
| **Egg, fried**         | 0  | 179  | trace   | 13.9  | 160       |
| **Egg, poached**       | 0  | 147  | trace   | 10.8  | 140       |
| **Egg, scrambled**     | 0  | 160  | trace   | 11.6  | 150       |
| **Egg white, raw**     | 0  | 36   | trace   | trace | 190       |
| **Egg, chicken, raw**  | 0  | 151  | trace   | 11.1  | 140       |
| **Egg, duck, raw**     | 0  | 163  | trace   | 11.8  | 120       |
| **Omelette, cheese**   | 0  | 271  | trace   | 23.0  | 921       |
| **Omelette, plain**    | 0  | 195  | 0       | 16.8  | 1024      |

# CHEESES

Cheeses have a GI of 0. There is a great variety of them and they provide a good source of calcium. They do, however, tend to be high in fat and sodium – adding salt is an essential part of the cheese-making process, so there is no such thing as salt-free cheese.

Try to keep the fat, salt and calorie level down by not having nibbles of cheese when you go to the fridge. Buy a variety that you really like and keep it as a treat and for use in cooking.

| | GI | kcal | Carbs g | Fat g | Sodium mg |
|---|---|---|---|---|---|
| **Brie** | 0 | 343 | 0 | 29.1 | 556 |
| **Caerphilly** | 0 | 373 | 0 | 31.3 | 500 |
| **Camembert** | 0 | 290 | 0 | 22.7 | 605 |
| **Cheddar** | 0 | 416 | 0.1 | 32.7 | 723 |
| **Cheddar, half-fat** | 0 | 273 | 0 | 15.8 | 670 |
| **Cheddar, vegetarian** | 0 | 390 | 0 | 32.0 | 670 |
| **Cheshire** | 0 | 381 | 0.1 | 31.8 | 502 |
| **Cottage cheese** | 0 | 101 | 3.1 | 3.9 | 300 |
| **Cottage cheese, reduced fat** | 0 | 79 | 3.3 | 1.5 | 300 |
| **Cream cheese** | 0 | 439 | 0 | 47.5 | 300 |
| **Danish Blue** | 0 | 342 | 0 | 28.9 | 1220 |
| **Double Gloucester** | 0 | 411 | 0.1 | 34.5 | 687 |
| **Edam** | 0 | 341 | 0 | 24.5 | 996 |
| **Edam, half-fat** | 0 | 229 | 0 | 10.9 | no figure |
| **Emmental** | 0 | 364 | trace | 28.0 | no figure |
| **Feta** | 0 | 250 | 1.5 | 20.2 | 1440 |
| **Goat's milk cheese** | 0 | 320 | 1 | 25.8 | 601 |

| | GI | kcal | Carbs g | Fat g | Sodium mg |
|---|---|---|---|---|---|
| **Gouda** | 0 | 377 | 0 | 30.6 | 925 |
| **Halloumi** | 0 | 316 | 1.6 | 24.7 | no figure |
| **Jaarlsberg** | 0 | 362 | 0 | 28 | 600 |
| **Lancashire** | 0 | 371 | 0 | 31.0 | 600 |
| **Leerdamer** | 0 | 358 | 0.1 | 28 | 870 |
| **Maasdam** | 0 | 343 | 0 | 27 | 500 |
| **Mascarpone, average** | 0 | 437 | 4.1 | 43.6 | no figure |
| **Mozzarella** | 0 | 257 | 0 | 20.3 | 395 |
| **Parmagiano reggiano** | 0 | 384 | 0 | 28 | 800 |
| **Parmesan** | 0 | 415 | 0.9 | 29.7 | 756 |
| **Red Leicester** | 0 | 411 | 0.1 | 34.5 | 687 |
| **Ricotta** | 0 | 134 | 2 | 10 | 100 |
| **Roulé** | 0 | 291 | 4.7 | 27.1 | 730 |
| **Smoked, processed** | 0 | 303 | 0.2 | 24.5 | 1270 |
| **Stilton** | 0 | 410 | 0.1 | 34.0 | 788 |
| **Talleggio** | 0 | 297 | 0 | 25 | 800 |
| **Wensleydale** | 0 | 380 | trace | 31.5 | 500 |

# DAIRY PRODUCTS

**including soya alternatives**

These all have a low GI and are a valuable source of calcium and protein. The milks provide a good base for drinks, sauces and bakes and can also be sipped alone – they are especially useful as a relaxing bedtime beverage. Keep an eye on the fat and calorie count, though.

For anyone with an intolerance to milk, soya alternatives can be substituted for cow's milk on cereal, in hot drinks or in recipes.

| | GI | kcal | Carbs g | Fat g | Sodium mg |
|---|---|---|---|---|---|
| **Alpro dairy-free alternative to milk, added calcium** | 32 | 46 | 2.6 | 2.2 | 56 |
| **Alpro dairy-free alternative to chocolate milk** | 37 | 81 | 10.7 | 2.4 | 55 |
| **Alpro chocolate dessert** | 52 | 87 | 13.6 | 2.3 | 55 |
| **Alpro vanilla dessert** | 47 | 80 | 12.7 | 1.8 | 53 |
| **Alpro strawberry yogurt** | 29 | 83 | 11.5 | 2.2 | 65 |
| **Butter, salted** | 0 | 744 | 0.6 | 82.2 | 606 |
| **Butter, unsalted** | 0 | 744 | 0.6 | 82.2 | 0 |
| **Condensed milk** | 61 | 333 | 55.5 | 10.1 | 140 |
| **Custard powder made with skimmed milk** | 35 | 95 | 16.4 | 2.0 | 67 |
| **Custard powder made with whole milk** | 35 | 118 | 16.2 | 4.5 | 67 |
| **Ice cream, chocolate, 15% fat** | 37 | 215 | 16.8 | 15.1 | 60 |
| **Ice cream, low-fat** | 50 | 119 | 13.7 | 6.0 | no figure |
| **Ice cream, full-fat** | 61 | 177 | 19.8 | 8.6 | 60 |
| **Ice cream, luxury** | 37 | 210 | 26 | 9.5 | no figure |
| **Milk drink – complete meal type** | 41 | 92 | 11.9 | 1.5 | 92 |

| | GI | kcal | Carbs g | Fat g | Sodium mg |
|---|---|---|---|---|---|
| **Milk, semi-skimmed** | 32 | 46 | 4.7 | 1.7 | 43 |
| **Milk, skimmed** | 32 | 32 | 4.4 | 0.3 | 44 |
| **Milk, soya** | 36 | 32 | 0.5 | 1.6 | 32 |
| **Milk, whole** | 31 | 66 | 4.5 | 3.9 | 43 |
| **Yogurt, low-fat** | 33 | 56 | 7.4 | 1.0 | 63 |
| **Yogurt, low-fat fruit** | 31 | 78 | 13.7 | 1.1 | 62 |
| **Yogurt, low-fat with sugar** | 33 | 56 | 7.4 | 1.0 | 63 |
| **Yogurt, soya** | 50 | 72 | 12.9 | 1.8 | 24 |
| **Yogurt, virtually fat free/diet plain** | 20 | 54 | 8.2 | 0.2 | 71 |
| **Yogurt drink** | 31 | 62 | 13.1 | trace | 47 |
| **Yogurt drink, probiotic** | 46 | 87 | 16 | 0.9 | trace |

# OILS, BUTTERS, MARGARINES & SPREADS

As these are mainly fat they all have a GI of 0. They are all high in calories, so enjoy them as a spread or in cooking but limit their use and use good quality oils for flavour. Try rapeseed or olive oil in cooking for flavour and for the mono-unsaturates they contain.

| | GI | kcal | Carbs g | Fat g | Sodium mg |
|---|---|---|---|---|---|
| **Butter, reduced fat** | 0 | 368 | 1.2 | 39.4 | no figure |
| **Butter, salted** | 0 | 744 | 0.6 | 82.2 | 606 |
| **Butter, spreadable** | 0 | 745 | trace | 82.5 | 390 |
| **Butter, unsalted** | 0 | 744 | 0.6 | 82.2 | 0 |
| **Cocoa butter** | 0 | 896 | 0 | 99.5 | 0 |
| **Coconut oil** | 0 | 899 | 0 | 99.9 | trace |
| **Corn oil** | 0 | 899 | 0 | 99.9 | trace |
| **Dripping, beef** | 0 | 891 | trace | 99.0 | 5 |
| **Ghee** | 0 | 895 | 0 | 99.4 | 1 |
| **Ground nut oil** | 0 | 824 | 0 | 91.6 | 100 |
| **Lard** | 0 | 891 | 0 | 99.9 | 2 |
| **Low-fat spread, 75% fat** | 0 | 680 | 0 | 75.5 | 1060 |
| **Low-fat spread, 40% fat** | 0 | 390 | 0.4 | 39.6 | 510 |
| **Margarine** | 0 | 718 | 1 | 81.6 | 800 |
| **Olive oil** | 0 | 899 | 0 | 99.9 | trace |
| **Olive spread, 21% olive oil** | 0 | 534 | 0 | 59.0 | 600 |
| **Palm oil** | 0 | 899 | 0 | 99.9 | trace |

|  | GI | kcal | Carbs g | Fat g | Sodium mg |
|---|---|---|---|---|---|
| **Pâté, liver** | 0 | 348 | 0.8 | 32.7 | 750 |
| **Pâté, mackerel** | 0 | 368 | 1.3 | 34.4 | 730 |
| **Pâté, tuna** | 0 | 236 | 0.4 | 18.6 | 390 |
| **Pâté, vegetable** | 0 | 173 | 5.9 | 13.4 | 540 |
| **Peanut oil** | 0 | 899 | 0 | 99.9 | trace |
| **Polyunsaturated spread, 20-25% fat** | 0 | 183 | 0.8 | 20 | 500 |
| **Polyunsaturated spread, 35-40% fat** | 0 | 365 | 1.8 | 41.5 | 650 |
| **Polyunsaturated spread, 70% fat** | 0 | 622 | 0.8 | 68.5 | 800 |
| **Rapeseed oil** | 0 | 899 | 0 | 99.9 | trace |
| **Sesame oil** | 0 | 899 | 0 | 99.7 | 2 |
| **Soya oil** | 0 | 899 | 0 | 99.9 | trace |
| **Spray oil** | 0 | 498 | 0 | 55.2 | 0 |
| **Sunflower seed oil** | 0 | 899 | 0 | 99.9 | trace |
| **Vegetable oil** | 0 | 899 | 0 | 99.9 | trace |
| **Walnut oil** | 0 | 899 | 0 | 99.9 | trace |

# PASTA, NOODLES, RICE & GRAINS

These are all considered to be starchy carbohydrate foods which we should be eating as the basis of all our meals. Their GI values vary a great deal, so try to choose those with a lower GI, such as basmati rather than white rice.

Add pearl barley or quinoa to soups and casseroles to lower the overall GI.

Have satisfying milk puddings like semolina pudding as desserts.

|  | GI | kcal | Carbs g | Fat g | Sodium mg |
|---|---|---|---|---|---|
| **Barley, pearl, boiled** | 25 | 120 | 27.6 | 0.6 | 1 |
| **Buckwheat, boiled** | 54 | 364 | 84.9 | 1.5 | 1 |
| **Couscous, cooked** | 65 | 227 | 51.3 | 1.0 | no figure |
| **Egg noodles, boiled** | 57 | 62 | 13 | 0.5 | 15 |
| **Egg noodles, fried** | 46 | 147 | 11.3 | 11.5 | 84 |
| **Fettucine** | 40 | 264 | 47.4 | 2.9 | 80 |
| **Gnocchi** | 68 | 152 | 33.6 | 0.3 | 600 |
| **Linguine, boiled** | 52 | 150 | 30.1 | 0.7 | 45 |
| **Macaroni, boiled** | 47 | 86 | 18.5 | 0.5 | 1 |
| **Pasta shapes, spiral** | 43 | 86 | 18.5 | 0.1 | 1 |
| **Quinoa** | 53 | 309 | 55.7 | 5.0 | 61 |
| **Rice, arborio, cooked** | 69 | 138 | 30.9 | 1.3 | 1 |
| **Rice, basmati, boiled** | 58 | 138 | 30.9 | 1.3 | 1 |
| **Rice, basmati, microwaved** | 52 | 116 | 24.9 | 1.2 | 100 |
| **Rice, brown, boiled** | 70 | 141 | 32.1 | 1.1 | 1 |
| **Rice, long-grain, boiled** | 56 | 138 | 30.9 | 1.3 | 1 |
| **Rice, long-grain, microwaved** | 52 | 116 | 24.9 | 1.2 | 100 |

| | GI | kcal | Carbs g | Fat g | Sodium mg |
|---|---|---|---|---|---|
| **Rice, long grain & wild** | 58 | 138 | 30.9 | 1.3 | 1 |
| **Rice, white, cooked** | 98 | 138 | 30.9 | 1.3 | 1 |
| **Semolina, creamy** | 55 | 79 | 12.6 | 1.7 | 100 |
| **Spaghetti, white, cooked** | 38 | 104 | 22.2 | 0.7 | trace |
| **Spaghetti, brown, cooked** | 37 | 113 | 23.2 | 0.9 | 45 |
| **Taco shells** | 68 | 506 | 61 | 23.0 | no figure |
| **Tapioca, creamy** | 81 | 75 | 12.4 | 1.8 | 100 |
| **Tortellini, cheese** | 50 | 183 | 25.5 | 5.1 | 100 |
| **Vermicelli, cooked** | 35 | 160 | 32.9 | 0.8 | 45 |

# BEANS, PEAS & LENTILS

These all have a low GI and are something to stock up the cupboard with. They are easily available and inexpensive. Many people are not sure about how to use them, but in fact lentils are easily cooked. A handful of dried lentils added to a curry or casserole helps to thicken the dish as well as holding the flavours in a rich thick sauce.

Dried beans need to be soaked overnight and some – particularly red kidney beans – need to be boiled thoroughly to destroy toxins. Purchasing the tinned varieties cuts out this hassle, but try to choose ones with reduced salt. If these are not available, give the salted beans a good rinse under running water.

Beans are good in salads as well as hot dishes and a can of mixed bean salad is a good and easy standby for bulking out a healthy meal.

| | GI | kcal | Carbs g | Fat g | Sodium mg |
|---|---|---|---|---|---|
| **Baked beans** | 48 | 84 | 15.3 | 0.6 | 530 |
| **Baked beans, reduced sugar & salt** | 48 | 73 | 12.5 | 0.6 | 330 |
| **Beansprouts** | 1 | 31 | 4 | 0.5 | 5 |
| **Black-eyed beans, soaked & boiled** | 42 | 116 | 19.9 | 0.7 | 5 |
| **Broad beans, fresh** | 79 | 59 | 7.2 | 1.0 | 1 |
| **Butter beans, tinned & drained** | 36 | 77 | 13 | 0.5 | 420 |
| **Butter beans, dried & cooked** | 31 | 103 | 18.4 | 0.6 | 9 |
| **Buckwheat, boiled** | 54 | 364 | 84.9 | 1.5 | 1 |
| **Chickpeas, dried & boiled** | 28 | 121 | 18.2 | 2.1 | 5 |
| **Chickpeas, tinned** | 42 | 115 | 16.1 | 2.9 | 220 |
| **Green beans, raw** | 1 | 24 | 3.2 | 0.5 | trace |
| **Green beans, boiled** | 1 | 25 | 4.7 | 0.1 | 8 |
| **Haricot beans, tinned & drained** | 38 | 94 | 15.7 | 0.5 | 99 |
| **Haricot beans, dried & boiled** | 33 | 95 | 17.2 | 0.5 | 15 |
| **Kidney beans, tinned & drained** | 36 | 100 | 17.8 | 0.6 | 390 |

| | GI | kcal | Carbs g | Fat g | Sodium mg |
|---|---|---|---|---|---|
| **Kidney beans, dried & boiled** | 28 | 100 | 17.4 | 0.5 | 2 |
| **Lentils green, dried & boiled** | 30 | 105 | 16.9 | 0.7 | 3 |
| **Lentils green, tinned in salt water** | 48 | 64 | 10.2 | 0.4 | 400 |
| **Lentils red, dried & boiled** | 26 | 100 | 17.5 | 0.4 | 12 |
| **Mung beans, dried & boiled** | 39 | 91 | 15.3 | 0.4 | 2 |
| **Peas, frozen, boiled** | 45 | 69 | 9.7 | 0.9 | 2 |
| **Peas, dried & boiled** | 39 | 109 | 19.9 | 0.8 | 13 |
| **Pinto beans** | 45 | 85 | 15.1 | 0.5 | 400 |
| **Split peas, dried & cooked** | 32 | 126 | 22.7 | 0.9 | 14 |
| **Soya beans, cooked** | 20 | 141 | 5.1 | 7.3 | 1 |

# BREAD, CAKES & BAKERY ITEMS

These come in a range of GI levels due to the different types of flour used. Common ingredients such as margarine and eggs have 0 GI and therefore reduce the overall GI of the finished product. However, cakes of all types tend to be high in calories so are best reserved as treats if you are trying to watch your calorie intake.

Seeded breads are a good choice as they have the lowest GI levels, but breads and wraps are generally a useful food as they are filling. Just watch that you do not put lots of butter or spread on them. Often the seeded ones are so tasty they do not need anything adding.

| | GI | kcal | Carbs g | Fat g | Sodium mg |
|---|---|---|---|---|---|
| **Angel cake** | 67 | 380 | 55 | 15.5 | 500 |
| **Bagel, white** | 72 | 273 | 57.8 | 1.8 | 550 |
| **Baguette** | 95 | 263 | 56.1 | 1.9 | 616 |
| **Banana cake** | 51 | 257 | 46.9 | 7.4 | 286 |
| **Bread, brown** | 73 | 207 | 42.1 | 2.0 | 443 |
| **Bread, gluten-free** | 78 | 258 | 98 | 12 | 960 |
| **Bread, granary** | 61 | 237 | 47.4 | 2.3 | 545 |
| **Bread, oat** | 47 | 237 | 43.5 | 3.0 | 1200 |
| **Bread, rye, no grains** | 51 | 219 | 45.8 | 1.7 | 580 |
| **Bread, rye/pumpernickel with grains** | 41 | 219 | 45.8 | 1.7 | 580 |
| **Bread, sourdough rye** | 53 | 184 | 37 | 1.2 | 280 |
| **Bread, soya & linseed** | 41 | 252 | 29.8 | 10.1 | 300 |
| **Bread, sunflower** | 57 | 240 | 39.6 | 4.7 | 470 |
| **Bread, sunflower & barley** | 57 | 240 | 39.9 | 6.1 | 250 |
| **Bread, white** | 70 | 235 | 49.3 | 1.9 | 520 |
| **Bread, white, added fibre** | 68 | 230 | 49.6 | 1.5 | 450 |
| **Bread, white spelt flour** | 74 | 235 | 49.3 | 1.9 | 520 |
| **Bread, wholemeal** | 77 | 217 | 42 | 2.9 | 487 |

|  | GI | kcal | Carbs g | Fat g | Sodium mg |
|---|---|---|---|---|---|
| **Bread stuffing** | 74 | 97 | 19.3 | 1.5 | 420 |
| **Carrot cake** | 62 | 341 | 47.3 | 16.3 | 400 |
| **Chapatti** | 63 | 202 | 43.7 | 1.0 | 120 |
| **Chocolate cake** | 38 | 456 | 50.4 | 26.4 | 430 |
| **Croissant** | 67 | 373 | 43.3 | 26.0 | 419 |
| **Crumpet** | 69 | 177 | 38.6 | 0.9 | 720 |
| **Cupcakes** | 73 | 468 | 54 | 24.0 | 400 |
| **Doughnuts** | 76 | 336 | 48.8 | 14.5 | 180 |
| **Flan cake** | 65 | 320 | 65.7 | 4.5 | 1400 |
| **Fruit bread** | 47 | 187 | 38.9 | 2.6 | 92 |
| **Fruit cake** | 54 | 371 | 57.9 | 14.8 | 250 |
| **Melba toast** | 70 | 388 | 75.1 | 2.4 | 900 |
| **Mountain Bread Wraps, Barley** | 61 | 282 | 54.5 | 1.4 | 210 |
| **Mountain Bread Wraps, Corn** | 72 | 278 | 53.6 | 1.4 | 200 |
| **Mountain Bread Wraps, Oat** | 41 | 278 | 53.2 | 1.5 | 200 |
| **Mountain Bread Wraps, Organic Wheat** | 63 | 287 | 54.4 | 1.5 | 270 |

|  | GI | kcal | Carbs g | Fat g | Sodium mg |
|---|---|---|---|---|---|
| **Mountain Bread Wraps, Rice** | 63 | 278 | 53.7 | 1.4 | 210 |
| **Mountain Bread Wraps, Rye** | 58 | 282 | 53.3 | 1.6 | 200 |
| **Mountain Bread Wraps, White** | 53 | 282 | 54.9 | 1.4 | 230 |
| **Mountain Bread Wraps, Whole Wheat** | 76 | 282 | 53.7 | 1.6 | 264 |
| **Muffins, blueberry** | 59 | 355 | 42.7 | 18.2 | 400 |
| **Muffins, chocolate chip** | 53 | 385 | 52.3 | 18.2 | 254 |
| **Pancakes** | 67 | 302 | 34.9 | 16.3 | 46 |
| **Pancakes from mix** | 67 | 152 | 27.4 | 1.8 | 400 |
| **Pastry** | 59 | 451 | 46.8 | 28.1 | 400 |
| **Pitta bread, white** | 57 | 255 | 55.1 | 1.3 | 439 |
| **Pop Tart-type product** | 70 | 386 | 69 | 10 | 400 |
| **Pretzels** | 83 | 381 | 79.2 | 3.5 | 1720 |
| **Scones, plain** | 92 | 364 | 53.7 | 14.8 | 840 |
| **Sponge cake** | 46 | 467 | 52.4 | 27.2 | 326 |
| **Taco shells** | 68 | 506 | 61 | 23.0 | no figure |
| **Vanilla iced cake** | 42 | 490 | 52.4 | 30.6 | 360 |
| **Waffles** | 76 | 334 | 39.6 | 16.7 | 580 |

# BREAKFAST CEREALS

These provide a good start to the day and are quick and easy to prepare and eat. They are good with extra added fruit.

Porridge is particularly useful as a breakfast as, if made with water, it has a low GI and helps fight off those dangerous mid-morning hunger pangs. It can be prepared in a very few minutes in a microwave oven or pan.

|                                               | GI | kcal | Carbs g | Fat g | Sodium mg |
|-----------------------------------------------|----|------|---------|-------|-----------|
| **All Bran**                                  | 30 | 270  | 48.5    | 3.5   | 850       |
| **Bite-size wholegrain**                      | 71 | 411  | 76.1    | 9.8   | 700       |
| **Bran buds**                                 | 58 | 273  | 52      | 2.9   | 510       |
| **Bran flakes**                               | 74 | 330  | 71.2    | 1.9   | 800       |
| **Bran cereal, noodle-shaped**                | 34 | 270  | 44      | 1.8   | 295       |
| **Cheerios**                                  | 74 | 368  | 80.7    | 3.8   | 800       |
| **Coco Pops**                                 | 77 | 383  | 91.5    | 2.5   | 450       |
| **Cornflakes**                                | 77 | 376  | 89.6    | 0.7   | 1000      |
| **Crunchy Nut Cornflakes**                    | 72 | 405  | 91.6    | 3.5   | 600       |
| **Frosties**                                  | 55 | 381  | 94.6    | 0.6   | 600       |
| **Grape nuts**                                | 71 | 345  | 20      | 2.0   | 500       |
| **Muesli, Swiss**                             | 56 | 363  | 72.2    | 6.7   | 380       |
| **Oat bran**                                  | 55 | 345  | 49.7    | 9.7   | 50        |
| **Porridge instant, made with semi-skim milk**| 66 | 100  | 13.8    | 2.8   | 40        |
| **Porridge oats, made with water**           | 42 | 46   | 8.1     | 1.1   | 565       |
| **Puffed Wheat**                              | 80 | 321  | 67.3    | 1.3   | 4         |

| | GI | kcal | Carbs g | Fat g | Sodium mg |
|---|---|---|---|---|---|
| **Raisin Wheats** | 61 | 332 | 71.5 | 1.5 | 100 |
| **Rice cereal, plain** | 82 | 382 | 92.9 | 1.0 | 650 |
| **Rice Krispies** | 82 | 382 | 92.9 | 1.0 | 650 |
| **Shredded wheat** | 75 | 332 | 71.7 | 2.2 | 8 |
| **Special K** | 54 | 373 | 75 | 1.0 | 800 |
| **Vogel Ultrabran** | 41 | 259 | 45.3 | 1.8 | 0.1 |
| **Vogel VitaPro** | 52 | 298 | 41.6 | 2.1 | 0.1 |
| **Weetabix** | 69 | 352 | 75.5 | 2.0 | 270 |
| **Wholegrain cereal cluster** | 66 | 351 | 66 | 9.0 | 300 |

# SAVOURY SNACKS
**including crisps, nuts & seeds**

Snacks can be a useful part of the diet and valuable for keeping up energy levels. Children and active people especially need snacks to keep them going.

However, snacks can add to the excess intake of calories so choose them wisely. The lower GI ones will keep you from feeling hungry for longer.

| | GI | kcal | Carbs g | Fat g | Sodium mg |
|---|---|---|---|---|---|
| **Cashew nuts, plain** | 22 | 573 | 18.1 | 48.2 | 15 |
| **Cashew nuts, roast & salted** | 22 | 611 | 18.8 | 50.9 | 290 |
| **Corn chips** | 42 | 459 | 54.3 | 31.9 | 1130 |
| **Crisps (potato)** | 54 | 530 | 53.3 | 34.2 | 800 |
| **Olives in brine** | 0 | 103 | 0 | 11.0 | 2250 |
| **Peanuts, plain** | 14 | 563 | 12.5 | 46.6 | 2 |
| **Peanuts, roasted & salted** | 14 | 602 | 7.1 | 53.0 | 400 |
| **Peanuts, dry roast** | 14 | 589 | 10.3 | 49.8 | 790 |
| **Pecans** | 10 | 689 | 5.8 | 70.1 | 1 |
| **Popcorn, plain** | 55 | 593 | 48.7 | 42.8 | 4 |
| **Popcorn, microwaved** | 51 | 440 | 62.5 | 17.7 | 10 |
| **Pork scratchings** | 0 | 606 | 0.2 | 46.0 | 1320 |
| **Pretzels** | 83 | 381 | 79.2 | 3.5 | 1720 |
| **Rice cakes** | 82 | 374 | 81.1 | 3.6 | no figure |
| **Sesame seeds** | 0 | 598 | 0.9 | 58.0 | 20 |

# SPREADS & DIPS
**both sweet & savoury**

These foods usually have a low GI and can be used on bread and toast. Unfortunately some, such as the nut spreads and butters, do have a high calorie content. So enjoy them but not in massive amounts.

The yeast and meat extracts are low in calories but high in sodium so again use them sparingly.

|  | GI | kcal | Carbs g | Fat g | Sodium mg |
|---|---|---|---|---|---|
| **Chocolate nut spread** | 33 | 549 | 60.5 | 33.0 | 50 |
| **Jam, apricot, reduced sugar** | 55 | 123 | 31.9 | 0.1 | 20 |
| **Jam, strawberry** | 56 | 261 | 69 | 0 | 29 |
| **Honey** | 55 | 288 | 76.4 | 0 | 11 |
| **Honey, manuka** | 39 | 314 | 80 | 0 | 12 |
| **Hummus** | 6 | 187 | 11.6 | 12.6 | 670 |
| **Marmalade** | 48 | 261 | 69.5 | 0 | 64 |
| **Meat extract** | 0 | 179 | 3.2 | 0.6 | 4370 |
| **Pâté, liver** | 0 | 368 | 1.3 | 34.4 | 730 |
| **Pâté, mackerel** | 0 | 236 | 0.4 | 18.6 | 390 |
| **Pâté, tuna** | 0 | 173 | 5.9 | 13.4 | 540 |
| **Peanut butter** | 23 | 606 | 13.1 | 51.8 | 350 |
| **Yeast extract** | 0 | 180 | 3.5 | 0.4 | 4300 |

# SNACK MEALS & SOUPS

Due to the protein and fat content these generally have a low GI but are relatively high in calories.

Lentil or homemade vegetable soup makes a really good and satisfying meal, low both in calories and in GI.

|  | GI | kcal | Carbs g | Fat g | Sodium mg |
|---|---|---|---|---|---|
| **Beef pie** | 45 | 299 | 22.1 | 19.4 | 460 |
| **Consommé** | 0 | 12 | 0.1 | 0 | 530 |
| **Macaroni cheese** | 47 | 86 | 12 | 2.7 | 400 |
| **Pea soup** | 66 | 40 | 7.3 | 0.8 | 300 |
| **Pizza, cheese & tomato, thin crust** | 36 | 238 | 30.1 | 8.8 | 248 |
| **Pizza, cheese & tomato, deep pan** | 36 | 249 | 35.1 | 7.5 | 247 |
| **Pizza, cheese, thin & crispy** | 30 | 277 | 33.9 | 10.3 | 282 |
| **Pizza, vegetarian** | 49 | 216 | 29.6 | 6.9 | 241 |
| **Ravioli, meat-filled** | 39 | 75 | 7 | 0.5 | 300 |
| **Soup, lentil, tinned** | 44 | 39 | 6.5 | 0.2 | 450 |
| **Soup, minestrone, tinned** | 39 | 31 | 5.7 | 0.5 | 302 |
| **Soup, tomato, tinned** | 38 | 52 | 5.9 | 3.0 | 400 |

# VEGETARIAN FOODS

**These foods are likely to feature in a healthy vegetarian diet. Soya products are also listed here.**

| | GI | kcal | Carbs g | Fat g | Sodium mg |
|---|---|---|---|---|---|
| **Alpro dairy-free alternative to milk, added calcium** | 32 | 46 | 2.6 | 2.2 | 56 |
| **Alpro dairy-free alternative to chocolate milk** | 37 | 81 | 10.7 | 2.4 | 55 |
| **Alpro chocolate dessert** | 52 | 87 | 13.6 | 2.3 | 55 |
| **Alpro vanilla dessert** | 47 | 80 | 12.7 | 1.8 | 53 |
| **Alpro strawberry yogurt** | 29 | 83 | 11.5 | 2.2 | 65 |
| **Hummus** | 6 | 187 | 11.6 | 12.6 | 670 |
| **Peanuts, plain** | 14 | 563 | 12.5 | 46.6 | 2 |
| **Peanuts, roasted & salted** | 14 | 602 | 7.1 | 53.0 | 400 |
| **Peanuts, dry roast** | 14 | 589 | 10.3 | 49.8 | 790 |
| **Pecans** | 10 | 689 | 5.8 | 70.1 | 1 |
| **Quinoa** | 53 | 309 | 55.7 | 5.0 | 61 |
| **Sesame seeds** | 0 | 598 | 0.9 | 58.0 | 20 |
| **Soya milk** | 36 | 32 | 0.5 | 1.6 | 32 |
| **Soya yogurt** | 50 | 72 | 12.9 | 1.8 | 24 |
| **Tofu, steamed** | 1 | 73 | 0.7 | 4.2 | 4 |
| **Tofu, fried** | 1 | 261 | 2 | 17.7 | 12 |
| **Vegeburger, grilled** | 59 | 196 | 8 | 11.1 | 490 |

# CONDIMENTS, SPICES, HERBS, DIPS & SAUCES

Salt and items containing a high proportion of it, such as yeast and meat extracts, are high in sodium, so should be eaten sparingly. Instead use a variety of herbs and spices. Ideally the herbs should be fresh, but dried ones make an acceptable substitute. Try basil with fish, parsley chopped into mashed potatoes, oregano in fish cakes and ginger in puddings.

Most herbs and spices have a very low GI as they are used in tiny amounts. As discussed in the introduction (see page 9), you would have to eat a vast quantity of them in order to test them according to current standards.

| | GI | kcal | Carbs g | Fat g | Sodium mg |
|---|---|---|---|---|---|
| **Allspice, ground** | 0 | no figure | no figure | 8.7 | 77 |
| **Anise seeds** | 0 | no figure | no figure | 15.9 | 16 |
| **Apple sauce** | 38 | 64 | 16.7 | 0.1 | 2 |
| **Baking powder** | 0 | 157 | 37.8 | 0 | 11800 |
| **Basil, dried** | 0 | 251 | 43.2 | 4.0 | 34 |
| **Basil, fresh** | 0 | 40 | 5.1 | 0.8 | 9 |
| **Bay leaf, dried** | 0 | 313 | 48.6 | 8.4 | 23 |
| **Betel leaves, fresh** | 0 | 61 | 8.6 | 0.1 | 7 |
| **Caraway seeds** | 0 | no figure | no figure | 14.6 | 17 |
| **Chervil, dried** | 0 | 237 | 37.8 | 3.9 | 83 |
| **Chilli powder** | 0 | 0 | no figure | 16.8 | 1010 |
| **Chinese 5 spice powder** | 0 | 0 | no figure | 8.7 | 63 |
| **Chives fresh** | 0 | 23 | 1.7 | 0.6 | 5 |
| **Cinnamon, ground** | 0 | no figure | no figure | 3.2 | 26 |
| **Cloves, dried** | 0 | no figure | no figure | 20.1 | 240 |
| **Coriander leaves, dried** | 0 | 279 | 41.7 | 4.8 | 210 |
| **Coriander leaves, fresh** | 0 | 20 | 1.8 | 0.6 | 28 |
| **Coriander seeds** | 0 | no figure | no figure | 17.8 | 35 |

|                          | GI | kcal      | Carbs g   | Fat g | Sodium mg |
|--------------------------|----|-----------|-----------|-------|-----------|
| **Cream-based dip**      | 0  | 360       | 4         | 37.0  | 330       |
| **Cumin Seeds**          | 0  | no figure | no figure | 18.2  | 150       |
| **Curry powder**         | 0  | 233       | 26.1      | 10.8  | 450       |
| **Dill, dried**          | 0  | 253       | 42.2      | 4.4   | 210       |
| **Dill, fresh**          | 0  | 25        | 0.9       | 0.8   | 26        |
| **Dill seeds**           | 0  | no figure | no figure | 14.5  | 20        |
| **Fennel seeds**         | 0  | no figure | no figure | 14.9  | 88        |
| **Fenugreek leaves, fresh** | 0 | 35      | 4.8       | 0.2   | 76        |
| **Fenugreek seeds**      | 0  | no figure | no figure | 7.4   | 43        |
| **Garam masala**         | 0  | 379       | 45.2      | 15.1  | 97        |
| **Garlic powder**        | 0  | 246       | 42.7      | 1.7   | 19        |
| **Gelatine**             | 0  | 338       | 0         | 0     | 330       |
| **Ginger, fresh**        | 0  | 49        | 9.5       | 0.7   | 11        |
| **Ginger, ground**       | 0  | 258       | 60        | 3.3   | 34        |
| **Hummus**               | 6  | 187       | 11.6      | 12.6  | 670       |
| **Lemon juice**          | 42 | 7         | 1.6       | trace | 1         |
| **Liquorice powder**     | 0  | no figure | no figure | 1.7   | no figure |
| **Mace, ground**         | 0  | no figure | no figure | 32.4  | 80        |

| | GI | kcal | Carbs g | Fat g | Sodium mg |
|---|---|---|---|---|---|
| **Marjoram, dried** | 0 | 71 | 42.5 | 7.0 | 77 |
| **Mayonnaise** | 0 | 691 | 1.7 | 75.6 | 450 |
| **Meat extract** | 0 | 179 | 3.2 | 0.6 | 4370 |
| **Mint, dried** | 0 | 279 | 34.6 | 4.6 | 98 |
| **Mint, fresh** | 1 | 43 | 5.3 | 0.7 | 15 |
| **Mixed herbs, dried** | 0 | 261 | 36.3 | 8.5 | 81 |
| **Mustard, made-up wholegrain** | 1 | 140 | 4.2 | 10.2 | 1620 |
| **Mustard powder** | 0 | 452 | 20.7 | 45.1 | 5 |
| **Nutmeg, ground** | 0 | 0 | no figure | 36.3 | 16 |
| **Oregano, dried** | 0 | 306 | 49.5 | 10.3 | 15 |
| **Oregano, fresh** | 0 | 66 | 9.7 | 2.0 | 3 |
| **Paprika** | 0 | 289 | 34.9 | 13.0 | 34 |
| **Parsley, dried** | 0 | 181 | 14.5 | 7.0 | 180 |
| **Parsley, fresh** | 0 | 34 | 2.7 | 1.3 | 33 |
| **Pepper, black** | 0 | 0 | no figure | 3.3 | 44 |
| **Pepper, cayenne, ground** | 0 | 318 | 31.7 | 17.3 | 30 |
| **Pepper, white** | 0 | 0 | no figure | 2.1 | 5 |

| | GI | kcal | Carbs g | Fat g | Sodium mg |
|---|---|---|---|---|---|
| **Poppy seeds** | 0 | no figure | no figure | 44.0 | 21 |
| **Rosemary dried** | 0 | 331 | 46.4 | 15.2 | 50 |
| **Rosemary fresh** | 0 | 99 | 13.5 | 4.4 | 15 |
| **Saffron** | 0 | 310 | 61.5 | 5.9 | 150 |
| **Sage dried** | 0 | 315 | 42.7 | 12.7 | 11 |
| **Sage fresh** | 0 | 119 | 15.6 | 4.6 | 4 |
| **Salt** | 0 | 0 | 0 | 0 | 39300 |
| **Salt, reduced sodium** | 0 | 0 | 0 | 0 | 13100 |
| **Soy sauce** | 1 | 43 | 8.2 | trace | 7120 |
| **Stock, chicken, home-made (average)** | 0 | 16 | 0.1 | 0.1 | 16300 |
| **Stock cube, chicken** | 1 | 237 | 9.9 | 15.4 | 16300 |
| **Stock cube, vegetable** | 1 | 253 | 11.6 | 17.3 | 16800 |
| **Stuffing, sage & onion** | 74 | 269 | 29 | 15.1 | 496 |
| **Tamarind leaves, fresh** | 0 | 115 | 18.2 | 2.1 | no figure |
| **Tarragon, dried** | 0 | 295 | 42.8 | 7.2 | 62 |
| **Tarragon, fresh** | 0 | 49 | 6.3 | 1.1 | 9 |
| **Thyme, dried** | 0 | 276 | 45.3 | 7.4 | 55 |

| | GI | kcal | Carbs g | Fat g | Sodium mg |
|---|---|---|---|---|---|
| **Thyme, fresh** | 0 | 95 | 15.1 | 2.5 | 18 |
| **Turmeric, ground** | 0 | no figure | no figure | 7.0 | 31 |
| **Stuffing sage & onion** | 74 | 269 | 29 | 15.1 | 496 |
| **Vinegar** | 0 | 22 | 0.6 | 0 | 5 |
| **Vinegar, balsamic** | 0 | 3 | 0.6 | 0 | no figure |
| **Vinegar, white wine** | 0 | 21 | 0.3 | 0 | 100 |
| **Worcester sauce** | 1 | 65 | 15.5 | 0.1 | 1200 |
| **Yeast extract** | 0 | 180 | 3.5 | 0.4 | 4300 |

# BISCUITS & CRACKERS

In general these have a high GI. Therefore make sure that you have a couple as a snack and not a packetful.

Oat biscuits have a lower GI than most, so are generally a good choice.

| | GI | kcal | Carbs g | Fat g | Sodium mg |
|---|---|---|---|---|---|
| **Arrowroot** | 65 | 472 | 76.7 | 15.2 | 500 |
| **Cereal bar** | 72 | 419 | 64.7 | 16.4 | 110 |
| **Corn cookies** | 87 | 382 | 70.9 | 3.1 | 259 |
| **Cream crackers** | 65 | 444 | 10 | 14.5 | 300 |
| **Digestive biscuits** | 59 | 465 | 68.6 | 20.3 | 600 |
| **Fruit bars** | 90 | 32 | 74 | no figure | no figure |
| **Gluten-free biscuits** | 58 | 461 | 72 | 17 | no figure |
| **Gluten-free crackers** | 87 | 480 | 58 | 23 | no figure |
| **Morning coffee** | 79 | 454 | 62.2 | 21.8 | 360 |
| **Muesli bar** | 61 | 376 | 64.3 | 10.1 | 100 |
| **Oatcakes** | 54 | 412 | 63 | 15.1 | 1230 |
| **Oatcakes, rough (Nairn)** | 33 | 429 | 57.1 | 17.7 | 700 |
| **Oatcakes, organic (Nairn)** | 28 | 423 | 70.2 | 16.0 | 700 |
| **Oatcakes, fine milled (Nairn)** | 48 | 448 | 53.7 | 21.1 | 700 |
| **Oatcakes, cheesey (Nairn)** | 55 | 476 | 45.5 | 26.7 | 1000 |
| **Oatcakes, mixed berry (Nairn)** | 36 | 433 | 68.9 | 13.9 | 400 |
| **Oatcakes, fruit & spice** | 39 | 424 | 64.6 | 14.9 | 300 |

| | GI | kcal | Carbs g | Fat g | Sodium mg |
|---|---|---|---|---|---|
| **Oatcakes, stem ginger** | 38 | 439 | 65.4 | 16.4 | 300 |
| **Rice cakes** | 82 | 374 | 81.1 | 3.6 | trace |
| **Rich Tea** | 55 | 427 | 74.8 | 13.3 | 410 |
| **Ryvita** | 63 | 332 | 58.6 | 6.0 | 400 |
| **Shortbread** | 64 | 509 | 63.3 | 27.5 | 270 |
| **Wafer biscuits** | 77 | 537 | 66 | 30.1 | 70 |
| **Water biscuits** | 71 | 440 | 75.8 | 12.5 | 470 |

# SUGAR & SWEETENERS

Sugar has a GI of 68 so is considered a medium GI food. While excess sugar is not good for teeth and also adds to calorie content, a little can be used for flavour and in cooking.

|  | GI | kcal | Carbs g | Fat g | Sodium mg |
|---|---|---|---|---|---|
| **Aspartame** | 0 | 392 | 95 | 0 | 0 |
| **Fructose** | 19 | 374 | 100 | 0 | 0 |
| **Fuisana Fruit Sugar** | 19 | 398 | 100 | 0 | 0 |
| **Glucose** | 100 | 375 | 100 | 0 | 0 |
| **Golden syrup** | 63 | 298 | 79 | 0 | 270 |
| **Lactose** | 43 | 375 | 100 | 0 | 0 |
| **Maple Syrup** | 54 | 262 | 67.2 | 0.2 | 9 |
| **Sucrose** | 68 | 394 | 100 | 0 | 5 |
| **XyloBrit 100% Xylitol** | 8 | 249 | 100 | 0 | 0 |

# DESSERTS & PUDDINGS

These always make a good end to a meal. Unfortunately they can also be a rich source of calories, sugar and fat. Many low-fat yoghurts and mousses have a low GI and make a healthier alternative. Sugar-free jellies are particularly useful as they are low in calories and fat; they can be varied by adding fruit and/or making them with skimmed milk or yogurt.

| | GI | kcal | Carbs g | Fat g | Sodium mg |
|---|---|---|---|---|---|
| **Blancmange** | 35 | 114 | 18.2 | 3.7 | 55 |
| **Berry mousse, 2.2% fat** | 36 | 101 | 11.1 | 1.5 | trace |
| **Chocolate mousse** | 31 | 149 | 19.9 | 6.5 | 67 |
| **Chocolate mousse, diet/low fat** | 37 | 123 | 18 | 3.7 | 69 |
| **Chocolate instant whip pudding** | 47 | 111 | 14.8 | 6.3 | 290 |
| **Egg custard** | 35 | 118 | 11 | 6 | 82 |
| **Ice cream, low-fat** | 50 | 119 | 13.7 | 6 | no figure |
| **Ice cream, full-fat** | 61 | 177 | 19.8 | 8.6 | 60 |
| **Ice cream, luxury** | 37 | 210 | 26 | 9.5 | no figure |
| **Jelly, fruit, sugar-free** | 0 | 6 | 0.1 | 0 | trace |
| **Sorbet** | 50 | 97 | 24.8 | 0.3 | 10 |

# SWEET SNACKS
**including sweets & chocolate**

Most of us love snacks, but sadly the majority are high in calories. Sweet snacks based on milk or yogurt are both low in GI and relatively low in calories.

However, if you are desperate, a few squares of chocolate or sweets should not do too much harm. The main thing is to keep it to a few and not demolish the whole family pack of sweets!

|  | GI | kcal | Carbs g | Fat g | Sodium mg |
|---|---|---|---|---|---|
| **Banana cake** | 51 | 257 | 46.9 | 7.4 | 286 |
| **Caramel-filled chocolate bar** | 62 | 473 | 77.3 | 18.9 | 150 |
| **Caramel & biscuit chocolate bar** | 44 | 492 | 68.5 | 25.4 | 190 |
| **Chocolate-covered nut bar** | 41 | 497 | 55.8 | 27.8 | 270 |
| **Chocolate-covered peanuts** | 33 | 520 | 60.2 | 28.7 | 1420 |
| **Chocolate, milk** | 49 | 520 | 56.9 | 30.7 | 85 |
| **Chocolate, plain** | 41 | 510 | 63.5 | 28.0 | 6 |
| **Chocolate, white** | 44 | 529 | 58.3 | 30.9 | 110 |
| **Chocolate mousse** | 31 | 149 | 19.9 | 6.5 | 67 |
| **Chocolate mousse, diet/low fat** | 37 | 123 | 18 | 3.7 | 69 |
| **Chocolate instant whip pudding** | 47 | 111 | 14.8 | 6.3 | 290 |
| **Digestive biscuits** | 59 | 455 | 68.6 | 20.3 | 600 |
| **Glucose sweets** | 100 | 375 | 100 | 0 | 0 |
| **Ice cream, low-fat** | 50 | 119 | 13.7 | 6 | no figure |
| **Ice cream, full fat** | 61 | 177 | 19.8 | 8.6 | 60 |

| | GI | kcal | Carbs g | Fat g | Sodium mg |
|---|---|---|---|---|---|
| Jelly beans | 78 | 370 | 90.3 | 0.4 | trace |
| Marshmallows | 62 | 327 | 83.1 | 0 | 29 |
| Milky filled chocolate bar | 44 | 445 | 74.8 | 15.8 | 100 |
| Nougat | 32 | 384 | 77.3 | 8.5 | 120 |
| Peppermints | 70 | 393 | 102.7 | 0.7 | 9 |
| Shortbread | 64 | 509 | 63.3 | 27.5 | 270 |
| Sponge cake | 46 | 467 | 52.4 | 27.2 | 326 |
| Vanilla iced cake | 42 | 490 | 52.4 | 30.6 | 360 |
| Yogurt, low-fat with sugar | 33 | 56 | 7.4 | 1.0 | 63 |
| Yogurt, virtually fat-free diet | 20 | 54 | 8.2 | 0.2 | 71 |
| Yogurt drink | 31 | 62 | 13.1 | trace | 47 |
| Yogurt drink, probiotic | 46 | 87 | 16 | 0.9 | trace |

# DRINKS alcoholic & non-alcoholic

We should all take at least 2 litres of liquid each day. This equates to 8 cups or glasses. Water is the ideal drink, whether straight from the tap, filtered or bottled. It provides no calories and has a GI of 0.

Sugar-free drinks and squashes all have a GI of 0 and coffees and teas with just a splash of skimmed or semi-skimmed milk will be between 4 and 5. Try to give up sugar in tea and coffee if you are watching the calories.

As explained in the introduction (see page 9) alcoholic beverages have not generally been tested for GI; but with the exception of beer, few of them contain carbohydrate, so they have a GI of 0. However, too much can damage the liver and they are a source of calories. The maximum healthy intake of alcohol is regarded as 21 units a week for adult women and 28 units a week for adult men (see box on page 22 for a definition of a unit). Also everyone should have at least one alcohol-free day each week.

| | GI | kcal | Carbs g | Fat g | Sodium mg |
|---|---|---|---|---|---|
| **Apple juice, unsweetened** | 40 | 38 | 9.9 | 0.1 | 2 |
| **Apple juice, unsweetened, clear** | 44 | 45 | 10.4 | 0.1 | 100 |
| **Apple juice, unsweetened, cloudy** | 37 | 49 | 11.9 | 0.1 | 100 |
| **Beer, bitter** | 110 | 30 | 2.2 | trace | 6 |
| **Bitter lemon** | 3 | 0 | 0.8 | 0 | 0 |
| **Brandy** | 0 | 222 | trace | 0 | trace |
| **Brown ale** | 110 | 30 | trace | trace | 16 |
| **Cappuccino** | 31 | 66 | 4.5 | 3.9 | 43 |
| **Chocolate hot drink sachet mix, made with water** | 51 | 78 | 4 | 2.4 | 200 |
| **Chocolate milk shake, semi-skimmed milk** | 41 | 69 | 11.3 | 1.6 | 52 |
| **Cider, dry** | 110 | 36 | 2.6 | 0 | 7 |
| **Cider, low alcohol** | 110 | 17 | 3.6 | 0 | 3 |
| **Cider, sweet** | 110 | 42 | 4.3 | 0 | 7 |
| **Coffee, black, no sugar** | 0 | 0 | 4.5 | 0 | 81 |
| **Cola** | 53 | 41 | 10.9 | 0 | 5 |
| **Cola, diet** | 0 | 0 | 0 | 0 | 5 |

|  | GI | kcal | Carbs<br>g | Fat<br>g | Sodium<br>mg |
|---|---|---|---|---|---|
| **Cranberry juice** | 52 | 61 | 14.4 | 0 | 0 |
| **Cranberry juice drink** | 56 | 48 | 11.5 | 0.1 | 100 |
| **Gin** | 0 | 222 | trace | 0 | trace |
| **Grapefruit juice, unsweetened** | 48 | 33 | 8.3 | 0.1 | 7 |
| **Herb teas** | 0 | 0 | 0.2 | 0 | 0 |
| **Lager** | 110 | 29 | trace | trace | 7 |
| **Lager, alcohol free** | 110 | 7 | 1.5 | trace | 2 |
| **Lager, low alcohol** | 110 | 10 | 1.5 | trace | 12 |
| **Lemonade, low-calorie** | 0 | 0 | 0.1 | 0 | 0 |
| **Malted milk drink, full-fat, with semi-skimmed milk** | 45 | 83 | 12.4 | 2 | 89 |
| **Nutrient-fortified drink** | 41 | 98 | 11.7 | 3.6 | 92 |
| **Orange juice, unsweetened** | 53 | 36 | 8.8 | 0.1 | 10 |
| **Orange, sparkling** | 68 | 18 | 4.4 | 0 | 0 |
| **Pineapple juice, unsweetened** | 46 | 41 | 10.5 | 0.1 | 8 |
| **Rum** | 0 | 222 | trace | 0 | trace |
| **Sherry, dry** | 0 | 116 | 1.4 | 0 | 10 |

| | GI | kcal | Carbs g | Fat g | Sodium mg |
|---|---|---|---|---|---|
| **Smoothie, raspberry** | 33 | 53 | 11.9 | trace | trace |
| **Soya drink – chocolate** | 34 | 71 | 10 | 1-7 | 60 |
| **Sparkling glucose drink** | 95 | 60 | 6 | 0 | 26 |
| **Sports drink** | 43 | 29 | 6.9 | trace | no figure |
| **Squash, made-up, sugar-free** | 0 | 4 | 1 | 0 | 8 |
| **Stout** | 110 | 30 | 1.5 | trace | 6 |
| **Tea, Chinese** | 0 | 1 | 0.2 | 0 | trace |
| **Tea, decaffeinated** | 0 | 1 | 0.2 | 0 | trace |
| **Tea, herbal** | 0 | 1 | 0.2 | trace | trace |
| **Tea, Indian** | 0 | trace | trace | trace | trace |
| **Tomato juice, no added sugar** | 8 | 14 | 3 | trace | 230 |
| **Vermouth, dry** | 0 | 109 | 3 | 0 | 11 |
| **Vodka** | 0 | 222 | trace | 0 | trace |
| **Water** | 0 | 0 | 0 | 0 | trace |
| **Whisky** | 0 | 222 | trace | 0 | trace |
| **Wine, red** | 0 | 68 | 0.2 | 0 | 7 |
| **Wine, white** | 0 | 66 | 0.6 | 0 | 4 |